Photodamaged Skin:
Clinical Signs, Causes and Management

Photodamaged Skin:

Clinical Signs, Causes and Management

Jean-Paul Ortonne, MD
Professor of Dermatology, Centre Hospitalier Universitaire de Nice, France

and

Ronald Marks, BSc, FRCP, FRCPath
Emeritus Professor, University of Wales College of Medicine, UK

Martin Dunitz

© Martin Dunitz Ltd 1999

First published in the United Kingdom in 1999 by

Martin Dunitz Ltd
The Livery House
7–9 Pratt Street
London NW1 0AE

All rights reserved. No part of this publication may be reproduced, stored in a retrieval system, or transmitted, in any form or by any means, electronic, mechanical, photocopying, recording or otherwise, without the prior permission of the publisher or in accordance with the provisions of the Copyright Act 1988, or under the terms of any licence permitting limited copying issued by the Copyright Licensing Agency, 33–34 Alfred Place, London WC1E 7DP.

A CIP catalogue record for this book is available from the British Library

ISBN 1 85317 345 2

Distributed in the United States by:
Blackwell Science Inc.
Commerce Place, 350 Main Street
Malden, MA 02148, USA
Tel: 1-800-215-1000

Distributed in Canada by:
Login Brothers Book Company
324 Salteaux Crescent
Winnipeg, Manitoba, R3J 3T2
Canada
Tel: 204-224-4068

Distributed in Brazil by:
Ernesto Reichmann Distribuidora de Livros, Ltda
Rua Coronel Marques 335, Tatuape 03440–000
Sao Paulo,
Brazil

Composition by Scribe Design, Gillingham, Kent

Printed and bound in Singapore by Kyodo Printing Co (S'pore) Pte Ltd

Contents

	Foreword	**vii**
1	Solar stimulus	1
2	Solar elastotic degenerative change	11
3	Dyspigmentation and melanoma	29
4	Photodysplasia and non-melanoma skin cancer	61
5	Intrinsic aging of skin	83
6	The effects of sun exposure on the immune response	97
7	The measurement of photodamage	109
8	The treatment of skin photoaging	121
	Index	143

Foreword

This is an exceedingly timely text. The cutaneous disorders in which sunlight plays a dominant or triggering role are very common and remarkably diverse with such a great variety of clinical expressions as to pose a diagnostic puzzle for the exprienced expert. Some photodermatoses are much more than skin diseases, having systemic concomitants which can threaten health and even life.

At the outset it should be noted that this book is not only comprehensive and thorough, it is also readable, lively and interesting. Scholarship is not sacrificed by the authors' humanistic style, as exemplified in opening statements:

> 'The sun and the energy it emits are the source of all life on earth. Its power is awe inspiring and was so wondrous to primitive peoples that it was often the central supernatural god figure in their system of religious beliefs. Despite the obvious benefits to agriculture and in supplying heat and light, sunlight is also a source of danger to animal life.'

It should also be noted that the two internationally recognized co-authors are examples of a breed which is in danger of becoming extinct, namely, the clinical investigator, who forms a bridge between basic science and clinical medicine. This interface is very evident in the way the authors deal with each disorder, extensively culling basic science reports from the literature, then blending these with the pertinent clinical features to create a balanced picture. Every chapter is richly referenced with thoughtfully selected papers, which can bring the interested student or researcher up to date without having to struggle through the hundreds of irrelevant random selections thrown up by Medline or Internet searches.

The co-authors are a happy duo who bring different perspectives to the subject owing to their geographic separateness; one having spent his professional life in the foggy climate of Wales (R.M.) and the other (J-P.) in the sun-drenched South of France.

Perhaps the most compelling reason for why this treatise should become a reference work for a variety of medical specialists is the remarkable demographic changes which have taken place in the last few decades, especially the aging of the population, known in the USA as the graying of America.

In affluent western countries, the proportion of elderly people over 65 is increasing rapidly. In fact, the greatest increase is in the segment past 85! The implications for the health and appearance of skin are profound. People have more time for recreational activities throughout the life span. Scant clothing exposes most of the body surface. People in cold northern climates can get to the sunniest areas, the Mediterranean for instance, within a matter of a few hours, where they can be burned to a crisp within 30 minutes. However, it is not the acute effects of heedless sun-exposure that is most devastating, painful as a sunburn is. Rather it is the delayed, chronic effects which wreak the greatest havoc. Most laymen are aware that the deterioration in facial features, previously called premature aging, is really the cumulative effect of years of heedless exposure to the sun, now appropriately called photoaging. Much more than appearance is involved since that same photoaged skin is the substrate for the development of benign and malignant neoplasms. Sunlight is an important contributing factor to malignant melanoma, a death-dealing disease whose prevalence has been doubling every 8 years.

The authors take all these lifestyle changes into account. They provide the theoretical base for understanding the complex processes of tumorigenesis. For example, the chapter on immunology focuses on how sunlight impacts on immune processes which influence carcinogenesis and the subsequent stages of tumor promotion and progression. Again, more than skin is involved. Patients who bear malignant tumors of the skin are at greater risk of internal cancers, probably due to impairment of immune defenses. The authors do not shy away from the daunting task of furnishing practical strategies for preventing and treating photodamaged skin, including the dramatic advances in laser surgery.

The genius of this book arises from its eclecticism. There is something here for every professional who has to deal with the good and bad effects of lifetime exposure to sunlight, *viz*, dermatologists, plastic surgeons, cosmeticians, aestheticians, pediatricians, geriatricians, and para-medical personnel.

Young mothers might also benefit from this crystal clear, informative account since they could constitute the forward echelon in the frustrating battle against the modern version of sun-worshipping and the craze for a *healthy* tan, an oxymoron to photobiologists.

Finally, there are still some people who do not know what dermatologists really do. This book is a testimonial to the far-reaching, activities mof well-trained dermatologists, the supreme generalists of skin, whose educational impact on all branches of biomedical science can no longer be ignored.

Albert M Kligman
University of Pennsylvania
1999

1 Solar stimulus

Introduction

The sun and the energy it emits are the source of all life on earth. Its power is awe-inspiring and was so wondrous to primitive peoples that it was often the central supernatural god figure in their system of religious belief. Despite the obvious benefits to agriculture and in supplying heat and light, sunlight is also a source of danger to animal life. This danger stems from the ultraviolet radiation (UVR) contained in the spectrum of solar energy and this chapter concentrates on this potentially damaging stimulus from the sun.

The amount of solar damage sustained by skin depends on the type and intensity of the solar irradiation, the opportunity for the irradiation to encounter exposed skin and the inherent susceptibility to damage from UVR of the individual concerned.

The solar spectrum

The sun is a blazing mass of hydrogen gas at the centre of the solar system that emits a continuous spectrum of energy which includes X-rays, γ-rays, radio waves, microwaves, visible light, infrared and ultraviolet radiations (Figure 1.1). Of major interest to dermatologists is the UVR segment of the radiation, as it is almost exclusively the cause of skin disorders arising from exposure to the sun. The UVR component of sunlight is composed of radiation with wavelengths of 200–400 nm and accounts for 8–9 per cent of the total energy emitted by the sun.[1] The UV region of the solar spectrum is further divided into several wavebands: UVA, UVB, UVC and vacuum UV in order of decreasing wavelength.[2] The UVA component is sometimes referred to as long-wave UVA, near UV or

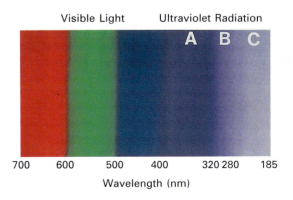

Figure 1.1

Complete solar spectrum.

black light, ranging from 320 to 400 nm. UVA is now subdivided into two photobiological regions: UVA1 between 320 and 340 nm, a waveband that has effects qualitatively similar to the nearby UVB waveband, and UVA2 ranging from 340 to 400 nm, which appears to involve distinctive oxygen-dependent photochemistry.[3] In energy terms the UVA radiation represents approximately 6.3 per cent of the sun's total emission.

The UVB waveband is about 1.5 per cent of the sun's total energy emission. This component is arbitrarily confined to those wavelengths below 320 nm, the cut-off point of ordinary window glass, and above 290 nm. UVB reaches earth in relatively small amounts, but is very efficient in promoting sunburn and pigmentation of human skin, hence the popular term for this part of the spectrum of the 'sunburn waveband'. It is also potentially very damaging to skin in the long term.

The UVC wavelengths (200–290 nm) do not reach the earth's surface as they are screened off by the upper atmosphere, including absorption by ozone formed photochemically in the stratosphere (Figure 1.2). Artificial UVC is strongly erythematogenic for human skin. So called vacuum UV is absorbed by air and does not play any role in cutaneous photobiology.

Visible light starts with blue light ranging through the colours of the rainbow to red and then on ultimately to infrared. The infrared radiation itself is often divided into near infrared (1–10 μm) and far infrared (>10 μm). Visible and infrared radiations represent 91.7 per cent of the incident sunlight energy.[1] Infrared radiation can cause significant skin damage leading to elastotic degenerative change of a distinctive type, with the alterations in the dermis taking place right throughout its depth, whereas the elastotic change due to UVR is for the most part confined to the upper dermis.[4]

A number of factors modify the ultraviolet component of sunlight at the earth's surface: the incoming beam of solar radiation is modified by scattering and absorption as it progresses through the atmosphere. Absorption by ozone is the dominant contributor to the absorption of UVC, such that radiation of wavelengths less than about 190 nm does not reach the surface of the earth. It also reduces the UVB component, but is a minor influence on the UVA component of terrestrial UVR.

The changing solar elevation in the heavens, and consequently the depth of the atmosphere through which the sun's rays have to penetrate to reach the earth, is highly variable, changing with latitude, the season and

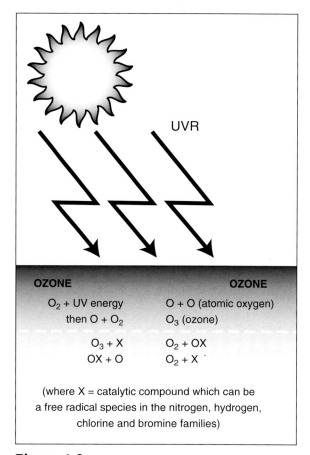

Figure 1.2

Ozone formation and ozone destruction by chlorofluorocarbons.

the time of the day and altitude, implying that the biosphere is exposed to a highly variable UVR energy field.

There is a fivefold reduction in erythemally effective UVB as one moves northwards from the tropics to northern Europe. The season of the year plays an important role with respect to intensity of UV radiation, especially as far as UVB is concerned. As an example, the sunburning effectiveness of sunlight in midsummer in northern Europe is about 130 times that of the sun at noon in midwinter. About 30–50 per cent of the total daily sunburning ultraviolet energy is received between 11 am and 1 pm. This means that most of the erythematogenic and carcinogenic UV rays reach the surface of the earth during this time of day. UVA exhibits much less variation with the time of the day. Backscattering by clouds attenuates the monthly mean UV irradiance to levels 50–80 per cent of the values expected for clear skies. Furthermore, monthly average irradiances can vary by 10–20 per cent from year to year just as a result of cloud cover[1] and the daily variations can amount to a factor of four. Other factors, such as clouds, surface reflection, wind, the relative humidity and the ambient temperature, are also important. Clouds attenuate the infrared components of sunlight more effectively than the UVR component. There may be more sunburning by the UVB around on a moderately cloudy day at midday even if it is cool, than on a clear day in the late afternoon.

Sand and snow, reflecting 25–30 per cent of the incident UVB radiation, may increase the exposure of unprotected areas of skin and may expose parts of the body that are normally not exposed. The same is probably true of white or grey concreted paths and pavements, and may explain why women seem especially prone to Bowen's disease of the lower legs and especially the shins (see page 70). Water is a good transmitter of UV radiation and it must be remembered that it is very easy to develop serious sun damage while swimming (or snorkelling). A series of experimental studies suggest that sunburn may be intensified by wind, that humidity increases acute UVR-induced skin damage and that the ambient temperature enhances both acute and chronic ultraviolet injury.

Sites below sea level are relatively poor in the UVB component of solar energy which reaches the earth's surface. This is well illustrated by the Dead Sea (400 m below sea level) where even prolonged sun exposure is not associated with sunburn and may explain the success of the Dead Sea 'spa' treatment of psoriasis. Conversely, each 300 m increase in altitude increases the sunburning effectiveness of sunlight by about 4 per cent.[5]

Several studies demonstrate that the natural UV radiation exposure depends upon the behaviour of the individual concerned. Outdoor workers receive greater personal UVR doses than indoor workers. The use of UV-sensitive films to measure the anatomical distribution of sunlight has shown that the areas of greatest sun exposure are the nose, the malar regions, the forehead and the top of the ear—areas where photodamage and non-melanoma skin cancer (NMSC) are very frequently observed.

Ozone

Ozone (or O_3) is a chemically reactive form of oxygen formed from molecular oxygen in the atmosphere by a photochemical reaction, the action of solar UVB on the oxygen it encounters. The oxygen formed in this way in the atmosphere would, if compressed, be approximately equal to a layer of about 3–4 mm thickness, although of course in nature ozone gas is dispersed throughout the entire atmosphere (although mostly between 15 and 50 km above the earth's surface at a parts per million concentration. Ozone has a vital function—it absorbs virtually all of the incident solar UVC as well as a goodly proportion of the incident UVB. Without this absorption by the ozone layer considerably more damaging UVR would reach the earth's surface than does at present. The effects of this would be spine-chilling: as a major consequence would be the death of the marine phytoplankton—the starting point of the sea's food chain. Ultimately human food resources would be threatened, as would all forms of terrestrial life. The enormous increase in skin cancer that would result if the ozone were suddenly to disappear would be the least of the problems that befall this planet.

Recent reports suggest that there have in fact been marked reductions of the amount of ozone present in the atmosphere, amounting to as much as 40 per cent over parts of Antarctica. The reduction in ozone is consequent to the release into the atmosphere of waste gases that attack the ozone molecule. A major source of these destructive emanations is the group of gases known as the chlorofluorcarbons (or CFCs). These 'inert' gases have been used extensively as propellants for sprays of different kinds, from paint to underarm deodorant, and have also been employed in the insulation, refrigeration, electronics and packaging industries. CFCs have the unfortunate property of hanging around in the atmosphere for a long period (reputedly 75–100 years). Their destructive capacity is the result of the interaction of CFCs with O_3 (Figure 1.2). Ammonia gas and nitrogen oxide are amongst the other gases that also have the effect of destroying atmospheric ozone.

The changes in the ozone content of the atmosphere due to man-made gases released into it are clearly of concern, but have nonetheless to be seen against the natural annual fluctuation, which can amount to 20 per cent of the total column of ozone.[1] Most of the data stem from observations made by the British Antarctic Survey team as well as by NASA, who have studied the problem in some depth. Their ozone trends panel have reported that not only is ozone thinning over heavily populated mid-latitudes in the order of 1–6 per cent per decade, but also that the trend is increasing.[6] Whatever the exact reduction in ozone levels it is quite plain that there is a consequent increase in UVB and an increase in the incidence of skin cancer. It has been computed that each 1 per cent increase in atmospheric ozone leads to an increase of about 2 per cent in 'consequences'. However, after 5 per cent loss the consequences are affected disproportionately so that a 10 per cent loss will result in a 24 per cent increase in consequences and a 30 per cent decrease will result in a 200 per cent increase in the consequences. Up until recently there was difficulty in detecting an increase in UVB at the earth's surface,[7] but a substantial increase was detected in Scotland in 1996 using sophisticated and automated spectrographic methods.[8]

Everything suggests that the increasing loss of ozone will result in increasing amounts of UVB reaching human skin and consequently an increased incidence of non-melanoma skin cancer (NMSC). It has been estimated from animal experiments that a 1 per cent decrease in atmospheric ozone will result in a 2 per cent increase in NMSC,[9] but at the time of writing it is not possible to say just how much skin cancer has already been caused by man's profligate destruction of ozone.

Massive attempts are being made by international bodies (e.g. the Montreal Convention) to stem the flow of destructive gases into the atmosphere.

Recent reports of stratospheric ozone depletion amounting to as much as 40 per cent over parts of Antarctica suggest that greater amounts of solar UVR will now reach the surface of the earth. It should be noted that a 1 per cent decrease in stratospheric ozone could cause about a 2 per cent increase in the amount of UVB that would pass through this shield.[7] Several studies have, however, failed to demonstrate an increase of UVB at ground levels between 1974 and 1985, suggesting that meteorological climatic and environmental factors in the troposphere may play an important role in attenuating UVB radiation, perhaps compensating for the ozone depletion.[7] Downward trends in the ozone layer in summertime at 45°N total only 3 per cent for the decade ending 1990. This change is small compared with a natural annual cycle of approximately 20 per cent in column ozone.[1]

Wavelength dependency of photodamage

Experimental data in animals and epidemiological data in human beings implicate the ultraviolet portion of sunlight, although infrared energy may also contribute. It is often argued that solar elastotic degeneration has to be caused by UVA, as only a little UVB penetrates into dermis (Figure 1.3). One study in the mouse,[10] demonstrating that skin photoaging is caused by UVA radiation only with a peak at 340 nm, supports this hypothesis. This study also concluded that other features of photoaging, such as glycosaminoglycan increase, collagen damage and wrinkling, are maximal with UVA irradiation. In other studies irradiation of mice with fluorescent UVA tubes only induced sparse elastotic change,[11,12] and other reports have concluded that UVB is a strong inducer of elastosis in mice.[12–14] One of them, using narrow-band UV radiation sources with emission peaks at 292, 300, 307, 317 and 336 nm, clearly demonstrated the dependence of solar elastosis in hairless mice on UVB wavelengths. The shorter the wavelengths the more pronounced was a subepidermal zone replacing the elastotic tissue of the deeper dermis.[15]

In fact, it seems more than likely that UVB and UVA may act synergistically. The reported induction of solar elastosis by long daily exposures to the Philips TL09 UVA tubes may be due to the concomitant emission of a substantial amount of UVB.[16] Stern

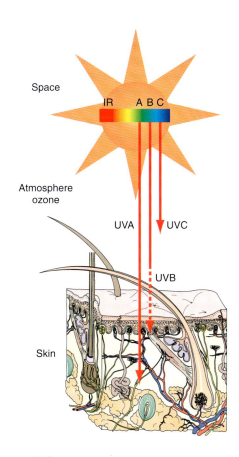

Figure 1.3

Ultraviolet radiation penetration into the skin.

et al suggest that the mild or moderate dose-dependent increase in photoaging occurring in patients receiving long-term psoralen plus ultraviolet A (PUVA) photochemotherapy may also be consequent on some UVB contamination.

Experimental data from action spectra studies in animals indicate that UVB is the most effective waveband in inducing cutaneous photodamage.[10,17,18] However, there is now evidence, also based on animal studies, that long-term irradiation with large doses of UVA can result in significant connective tissue damage[13] analogous to that associated with long-term sun exposure.[19] A recent study of the effects of repeated exposures to suberythemal doses of UVB and UVA in human skin shows that UVA induces greater cumulative changes than solar-simulated radiation. Histological examination revealed that repeated suberythemal doses of UVB and UVA in human skin showed that UVA induces greater cumulative changes than solar-simulated radiation. Lavker et al's study[20] revealed that repeated suberythematogenic doses of UVA were more effective than UVB in inducing stratum corneum thickening, epidermal hyperplasia, depletion of Langerhans' cells, inflammatory cell infiltrate in the skin and deposition of lysozyme on elastin fibres. These findings suggest that UVA may contribute significantly to long-term actinic damage.

The role of infrared radiation

Infrared radiation, which comprises about 40 per cent of solar radiation, has long been recognized for its harmful effects on the integument.[21] The condition of erythema ab igne results from chronic heating of the skin – usually the lower legs – and the histological changes seen, such as focal hyperkeratosis and dyskeratosis and elastic fibre hyperplasia, are nearly identical to those seen in photodamaged skin.[4,22] Interestingly, the elastotic degenerative change is found throughout the dermis in erythema ab igne (Figure 1.4). Presumably this is because of the much greater penetration of infrared compared with UVR. The contribution of infrared radiation to the pathogenesis of solar elastosis has also been discussed,[23] but not confirmed by experimental studies in mice.[24] Certainly chronic heat injury is a well-established course of NMSC.[25] Visible light is unlikely to have any pathogenetic role in the production of solar elastosis. The main

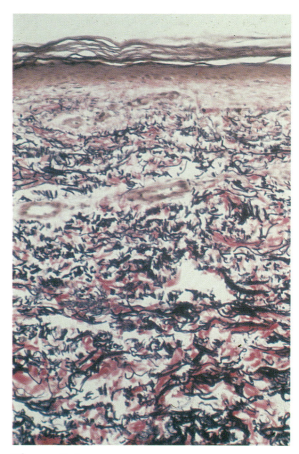

Figure 1.4

Elastosis throughout depth of dermis in erythema ab igne.

features in erythema ab igne suggest that infrared radiations may participate in the induction of some of the abnormal features noted in photodamaged skin. It has recently been demonstrated that repeated mild heating of the skin of volunteer subjects can result in epidermal thickening and hyperproliferation similar to changes seen after UVR.[26]

Socioeconomic and cultural considerations

Clothing

Clothing is a major factor influencing the dose of solar UVR received by the skin. The area of skin exposed depends partially on the climate but to a greater extent on the customs and fashion of the culture considered. Dress codes vary between ethnic and religious groups and are also dependent on the occupation and social standing of the individuals concerned and on the prevailing fashion. In much of the Middle East, North Africa and the Gulf States, photodamage and NMSC are fairly uncommon as it has been customary to expose very little skin on account of the prevailing customs and religious beliefs. In nearby Israel, however, where there is a similar climate but a different religious tradition and different customs, NMSC has become quite a public health problem.

The thickness and weave of textiles also influence whether significant amounts of solar UVR will reach the skin. It seems that the denser fabrics offer more protection than loosely woven materials. It is quite easy to develop sunburn whilst wearing a thin shirt or blouse, and in some countries a sun protection factor (SPF) is assigned to some fabrics and they are promoted on this basis. There is some debate as to whether all fabrics protect right across the UV spectrum. On balance it seems that textiles do not have specific filtering properties. Davies et al[27] have reviewed this complex topic and conducted studies on many different types of fabrics. They used a spectrophotometric method to assess protection and found that most white fabrics tested did not give an SPF of greater than 15. Polyester fabrics seem to be better than cotton, and coloured fabrics also provided more protection than white materials. Fortunately, laundering seems to have little effect on the assigned SPF of a fabric.[28]

Before leaving this topic mention should be made of the protection against the sun offered by stockings, as the lower legs of women seem curiously prone to development of NMSC. Sinclair and Diffey[29] concluded that the SPF increased for black stockings from 1.5 to 3 between 10 and 40 denier. The average stocking (15 denier) only provides the minimal protection of an SPF of about 2.

Outdoor activities

Occupation is a major determinant of the amount of skin exposure to solar UVR that occurs. Agricultural workers, building site operatives (particularly those who work on roofs), sailors and professional sportsmen and women are amongst those especially at risk.

Leisure activities are also quite major determinants of the total dose of solar UVR encountered by skin on an annual basis. In the past 50 years there have been major reductions in the numbers of hours worked per week. On average the British working week now is 37.5 hours and it is even less in some other countries of Europe. The entitlement to paid leave has also increased so that it is by no means uncommon for employees to have 4–6 weeks of holiday annually. Alongside this reduction in time commitment to work two other trends are important. The first of these is the growing affluence of the Western world which has left a substantial proportion of the population with both time and money on its hands. The other trend, which while undeniable remains difficult to quantify and impossible to justify, is the almost universal wish to appear suntanned. This appears to have started in the 1920s with the well-publicized exploits of the wealthy South of France 'set' and in particular the female fashion icon Coco Chanel. It seems that being brown from sunbathing was identified in the minds of the populace with pleasure, privilege and attractiveness and since then many ordinary citizens of European origin have tried to emulate the darker and browner skin tones because of this.

The package holiday industry has grown up in response to the increased time and money available and has been encouraged by the cult of sun worship and slick advertising. It has also been spurred on by the drop in the price of aviation fuel and the consequent reduction in the price of air travel. Literally millions of pale northern Europeans flood the coastal concrete jungles on the Mediterranean, Aegean, Caribbean and Adriatic coast lines – and sustain serious solar injury as a result. Sun-blessed areas further afield, including the East African coastline, South Africa, Thailand and northern Australia are not immune to this invasion of eager European holiday-makers. At one time in the UK a week at Blackpool was the expected and eagerly anticipated reward for a hard year's manual work. Such are the socioeconomic changes that have taken place in recent years that two or even more sun holidays per year are within the reach of many in the growing middle classes and a proportion of the skilled workforce. During the late 1970s the numbers of visits by UK residents travelling abroad and overseas residents visiting the UK were broadly similar, but in the 1990s the difference widened with nearly twice as many visits made by UK residents as by individuals from overseas. In 1993 16 per cent of British residents took two holidays. All this, while admirable as a historic improvement in lifestyle and living conditions, has meant a considerable increase in the average dose of UVR to the average British citizen.

A study from Norway has concluded that there was a highly significant association between melanoma incidence and the dose of UVB received and that the changes in incidence of melanoma between 1955 and 1969 and between 1985 and 1989 were significantly positively associated with holidays abroad.[30] In another 'pan-European' study[31] it was found that outdoor occupations carried a significantly greater risk for squamous cell carcinoma (odds ratio of 1.6 for 54 000 cumulated hours of exposure), whereas recreational exposure seemed to predispose specifically to basal cell carcinoma (odds ratio 1.6 for more than 2600 cumulated hours on holiday at the beach).

There can be little doubt that changes in social conditions, aspirations and cultural practices influence the dose of UVR received and have been a major reason for the worldwide increase in the incidence of skin cancer. Although it is intrinsically more difficult to collect data concerning photoaging, everything points to there being parallel changes in this sequel of chronic sun exposure as well.

References

1. Chapman RS, Cooper KD, De Fabo EC et al, Solar ultraviolet radiation and the risk of infectious disease: summary of a workshop. *Photochem Photobiol* (1995) **61**: 223–47.
2. Shea CR, Parrish JA, Non ionizing radiation and the skin. In: LA Goldsmith (ed.) *Physiology Biochemistry and Molecular Biology of the Skin*, Vol. 2, 2nd edn. Oxford University Press: Oxford, 1991, pp. 910–27.
3. Peak MJ, Peak JG, Carnes BA, Induction of direct and indirect single strand breaks in human cell DNA by far and near ultraviolet radiations: action spectrum of normal human skin. *Photochem Photobiol* (1987) **45**: 381–7.
4. Shahrad P, Marks R, The wages of warmth: changes in erythema ab igne. *Br J Dermatol* (1977) **97**: 179–86.
5. Diffey BL, Larko O, Clinical climatology. *Photodermatol* (1984) **1**: 30–7.
6. Lloyd SA, Stratospheric ozone depletion. *Lancet* (1993) **342**: 1156–8.
7. Scotto J, Cotton G, Urbach F et al, Biologically effective ultraviolet radiation: surface measurements in the United States 1974–1985. *Science* (1988) **239**: 762–4.

8. Moseley H, Mackie RM, Ultraviolet B radiation was increased at ground level in Scotland during a period of ozone depletion. *Br J Dermatol* (1995) **137**: 101–10.
9. Oumeish OY, The global ozone crisis. *Clinics Dermatol* (1998) **16**: 11–17.
10. Bissett DL, Hannon DP, Orr TV, Wavelength dependence of histological physical and visible changes in chronically UV irradiated hairless mouse skin. *Photochem Photobiol* (1989) **50**: 763–9.
11. Kligman LH, Photodamage to dermal connective tissue by UVA. In: F Urbach, RW Gange (eds) *The Biological Effects of UVA Radiation*. Praeger: New York, 1986, pp. 98–104.
12. Poulsen JT, Staberg B, Wulf HC, Brodthagen H, Dermal elastosis in hairless mice after UVA and UVB applied simultaneously separately or sequentially. *Br J Dermatol* (1984) **110**: 531–8.
13. Kligman LH, Akin FK, Kligman AM, The contribution of UVA and UVB to connective tissue damage in hairless mice. *J Invest Dermatol* (1985) **84**: 272–6.
14. Berger H, Tsambaos D, Mahrle G, Experimental elastosis induced by chronic ultraviolet exposure. *Arch Dermatol Res* (1980) **269**: 39–49.
15. Wulf HC, Poulsen T, Davies RE, Urbach F, Narrow band UV radiation and induction of dermal elastosis and skin cancer. *Photodermatol* (1989) **6**: 44–57.
16. Stern RS, Parrish JA, Fitzpatrick TB et al, Actinic degeneration in association with long term use of PUVA. *J Invest Dermatol* (1985) **84**: 135–8.
17. Cole CA, Forbes PD, Davies RE, An action spectrum for UV photocarcinogenesis. *Photochem Photobiol* (1986) **43**: 275–84.
18. Sterenborg HM, Van der Leun JC, Action spectra for tumorigenesis by ultraviolet radiation. In: WF Pacchier, BFM Bosnjakovic (eds) *Human Exposure to Ultraviolet Radiation: Risks and Regulations*. Elsevier: Amsterdam, 1987, pp. 173–9.
19. Kligman LH, Gebre M, Biochemical changes in hairless mouse skin collagen after chronic exposure to ultraviolet-A radiation. *Photochem Photobiol* (1991) **54**: 233–7.
20. Lavker RM, Gerberick F, Veres D et al, Cumulative effects from repeated exposures to suberythemal doses of UVB and UVA in human skin. *J Am Acad Dermatol* (1995) **32**: 53–62.
21. Dover JS, Phillips TJ, Arndt KA, Cutaneous effects and therapeutic uses of heat with emphasis on infrared radiation. *J Am Acad Dermatol* (1989) **20**: 278–86.
22. Finlayson GR, Sams WM, Smith JG, Erythema ab igne: a histopathological study. *J Invest Dermatol* (1966) **46**: 104–8.
23. Kligman LG, Intensification of ultraviolet induced dermal damage by infrared radiation. *Arch Dermatol Res* (1982) **272**: 229–38.
24. Wulf HC, Poulsen T, Davies RE et al, Narrow band UV radiation and induction of dermal elastosis and skin cancer. *Photo-Dermatology* (1989) **6**: 44–51.
25. Dover JS, Phillips TJ, Arndt KA, Cutaneous effects and therapeutic uses of heat with emphasis on infrared radiation. *J Am Acad Dermatol* (1989) **20**: 278–86.
26. Edwards C, Gaskell SA, Hill SA et al, The effects on human epidermis of chronic suberythemal exposure to pure infra-red radiation. *Arch Dermatol* (1998) In press.
27. Davis S, Capjack L, Kerr N et al, Clothing as protection from ultraviolet radiation: which fabric is most effective? *Int J Dermatol* (1997) **36**: 374–9.
28. Stanford D, Gergoura KE, Pailthorpe MT, The effect of laundering on the sun protection afforded by a summer weight garment. *J Eur Acad Dermatoven* (1995) **5**: 28–30.
29. Sinclair SA, Diffey BL, Sun protection provided by ladies stockings. *Br J Dermatol* (1997) **136**: 239–41.
30. Bentham G, Aase A, Incidence of malignant melanoma of the skin in Norway, 1955–1989: associations with solar ultraviolet radiation, income and holidays abroad. *Int J Epidem* (1996) **25**: 1132–8.
31. Zanetti R, Rosso S, Martinez C et al, The multicentre south European study 'Helios'. I: Skin characteristics and sunburns in basal cell and squamous cell carcinomas of the skin. *Br J Cancer* (1996) **73**: 1440–6.

2 Solar elastotic degenerative change (syn. solar elastosis)

Introduction

Skin that has been habitually exposed to the sun looks battered and old. It is this fact that inspired the term 'photoaging', which although apt, gives out the wrong message as it implies that sunlight has itself somehow caused aging. The clinical changes produced by solar elastosis are in fact only superficially similar to chronological aging and are almost entirely the result of damage sustained from long-term exposure to solar ultraviolet radiation (UVR). There can be little doubt that if you want to stay looking young you should stay out of the sun! Nonetheless it is true that the older one becomes the more photodamage one sustains merely because the natural skin repair processes are slow and the solar damage sustained accumulates.

In temperate climates such as those of north-west Europe the degenerative changes due to sun exposure may be detected histologically as early as in the second half of the third decade but are not usually visible clinically till the fourth decade is reached. This is not the case in tropical and subtropical climates. In discussion with Australian colleagues it becomes clear that in their experience severe chronic solar damage appears earlier in life and is of a different order of magnitude compared with the degree of damage usually found in Europe. Virtually all their patients show clinical signs that we would regard as being indicative of severe solar damage. Our suspicion that the greater the cumulated dose of solar UVR, the more the photodamage present was confirmed by a recent study from the USA.[1] It will be very interesting to see whether recent campaigns and warnings in the news media against prolonged sun exposure will make any difference to the amount or severity of sun damaged skin observed in the community.

Apart from the cumulated dose of solar UVR there are other factors that influence the degree of photodamage that develops on an individual's sun-exposed skin. The most important of these is the degree of skin pigmentation. Darkly pigmented individuals from Africa and Asia are much more protected than fair-skinned Europeans and the susceptibility to solar injury roughly parallels the Boston skin type classification (see Table 2.1). Pigment protection, however, is not absolute. Even the most heavily melanized individual can become sun-damaged if the dose of solar UVR is great enough. Other factors may also influence the development of photodamage, including the readiness with which the skin repairs itself after UV injury and other environmental influences such as the amount of concomitant solar infrared irradiation.

Table 2.1 Skin types and recommended sunscreen protection factor

Skin type	Sensitivity to UV	Sunburn and tanning history	Recommended sun protection factor
I	Very sensitive	Always burns easily; never tans	10 or more
II	Very sensitive	Always burns easily; tans minimally	10 or more
III	Sensitive	Burns moderately; tans gradually and uniformally (light brown)	8 to 10
IV	Moderately sensitive	Burns minimally; always tans well (moderate brown)	6 to 8
V	Minimally sensitive	Rarely burns, tans profusely (dark brown)	4
VI	Insensitive	Never burns; deeply pigmented (black)	None indicated

From: Pathak MA, Fitzpatrick TB, Preventative treatment of sunburn, dermatoheliosis and skin cancer with sun protective agents. In: TB Fitzpatrick (ed.) *Dermatology in General Medicine.* McGraw-Hill Inc, Vol. 4, 1993, p. 1684.

Interestingly, some ethnic groups seem predisposed to UVR injury of all sorts and although the basis for this is uncertain, deficient or slow repair may be part of the explanation for this predisposition. The Oklahoma Indians and the Celts are two such groups who are notorious for their susceptibility to photodamage of all types. The basis for this ethnic propensity[2] to sun damage is not clear. It is also discussed in Chapter 4. The bulk of the clinical changes observed in sun-damaged skin are due to alterations in structure and function of both the epidermis and the dermis, although most of the more obvious clinical abnormalities are due to the dermal changes. These are known as solar elastotic degenerative change or just 'solar elastosis' and are the focus of this chapter.

Clinical features of solar elastosis

The best known clinical feature of solar elastosis is wrinkling, but not all wrinkling is due to this kind of degenerative change. The major crease lines and furrows on the forehead and in the nasolabial grooves seem to be the result of a combination of gravity, 'habit', muscle laxness or spasm, and subcutaneous 'tissue failure'. Intracutaneous injections of botulinum toxin around the forehead and glabella crease lines and furrows reduce the prominence of these lines greatly and presumably they result in large part from muscle spasm. Solar elastosis seems to be the cause of the prolific fine lines on the face of sun-damaged individuals, which occur particularly around the mouth (Figure 2.1), on the cheeks (Figure 2.2) and at the sides of the eyes (a condition known colloquially as 'crow's feet'). The wrinkles result from the altered physical properties of the elastotic dermal connective tissue. One study using a variety of sophisticated measuring methods found that there was a strong relationship between the degree of solar elastosis and the extent of wrinkling on the one hand and the elastosis and the perceived age on the other.[3] The fine lines found around the mouth may at least in part be due to cigarette smoking, but the evidence is not conclusive at present.[4] A further typical clinical change due to solar elastosis is the development of a marked skin discoloration on the sun-exposed sites best described as a dull, lemon yellow to brown in hue (sometimes called citrine skin) or what is often described as 'sallow'. This is not seen at

Solar elastotic degenerative change

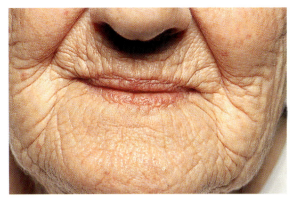

Figure 2.1
Fine lines around mouth due to photodamage in an elderly lady.

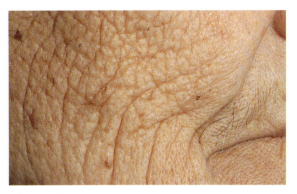

Figure 2.2
Fine lines on cheek due to photodamage in an elderly lady.

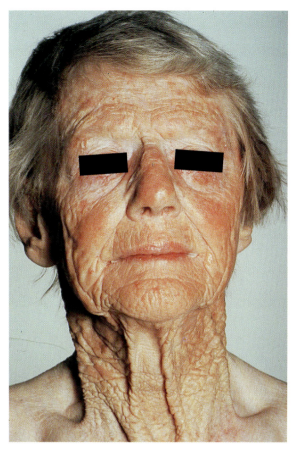

Figure 2.3
Yellowish discoloration of very photodamaged skin. This change is very noticeable on the neck.

all affected sites or in all individuals but is a common enough alteration (Figure 2.3). The cause of this odd alteration of skin colour is not yet explained. The affected skin may seem somewhat thicker than normal and may look leathery. Examination by pulsed A-scan ultrasound confirms the increased thickness of the abnormal dermis. B-scan ultrasound imaging reveals the presence of an echo-poor (echolucent) band immediately subepidermally that investigations have shown to be due to the absence of normal fibrillar collagen and the presence of the abnormal solar elastotic material (see page 21). In fact either 'A-scan' or 'B-scan' ultrasound can be used to determine the degree of elastotic degeneration present on the basis of this reduction in ultrasound echos in the affected areas.

Telangiectasia is often present in areas of solar elastosis. It is most noticeable over the nose, cheeks and chin, but may be seen anywhere on the facial skin (Figures 2.4 and

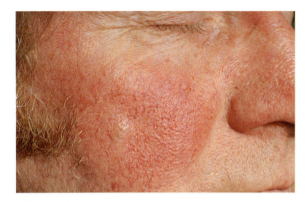

Figure 2.4

Redness and telangiectasia affecting the cheek as a result of photodamage.

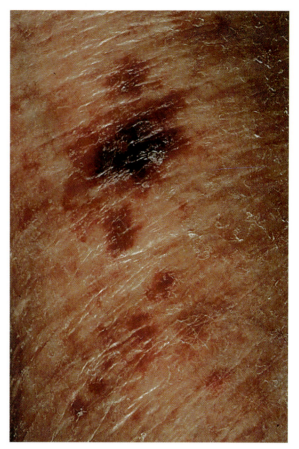

Figure 2.6

Senile (solar) purpura on the forearm of photodamaged subject.

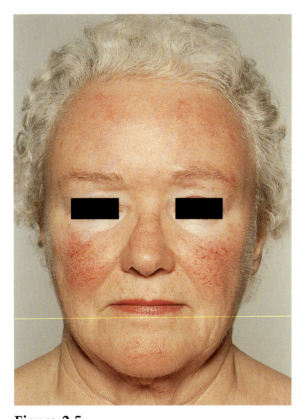

Figure 2.5

Redness and telangiectasia of the cheeks. Is this due to photodamage or erythemato telangiectetic rosacea?

2.5). In some individuals there is also a diffuse dull erythema of the cheeks, nose, neck and chin. Both the telangiectasia and the erythema are the result of loss of the normal dermal collagenous support to the superficial capillary vasculature and its replacement by abnormal mechanically inefficient elastotic tissue. This allows the small blood vessels to dilate passively. In some patients these vascular alterations are the most prominent clinical features and then it may be difficult to

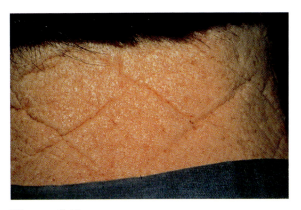

Figure 2.7
Cutis rhomboidalis nuchae in an elderly man.

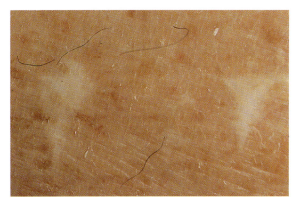

Figure 2.8
Triradiate (stellate) scars on the forearm of a photodamaged subject.

distinguish this persistent erythema from the clinical features of rosacea (Figure 2.5). As rosacea is predominantly a disorder of fair skinned individuals of north-west European ancestry in whom marked solar elastosis is evident histologically,[5] genuine difficulty arises in separating the two conditions. Senile purpura results from the exposure and vulnerability to mechanical trauma of the unprotected superficial vasculature (see later) (Figure 2.6).

Clinical variants of solar elastosis

Cutis rhomboidalis nuchae

The presence of a regular lattice of rhomboidal furrows on the back of the neck in fair skinned photodamaged middle-aged and elderly men is not uncommon (Figure 2.7). The background reddish colour to this dramatically deformed sun-damaged skin and the condition's frequency explain the colloquial North-American term 'Red neck' for any fair-skinned agricultural or other type of outdoor worker from the 'sun belt'. Another colloquial name for the condition, 'sailor's skin', reflects the high frequency of the disorder in seamen exposed to the elements as part of their job. Sailing now seems to have more to do with the understanding of computers rather than with hauling on ropes and chains and probably the condition will be less frequent in future. The deep furrows at the back of the neck are likely to be the result of the altered mechanical properties of the elastotic skin (see below), as are facial wrinkles, but the reason for the curious rhomboidal pattern is unclear. It seems to be the signature of skin that is often put on the stretch, as for example the skin around joints, whose skin surface pattern is rhomboidal.

Pseudocolloid milium

This curious condition is really no more than very severe solar elastosis localized to a small area of skin. Localized yellowish-white papules and plaques 2–3 cm in diameter appear in the most sun-exposed skin sites, such as the backs of the hands and forearms and the malar regions of the cheeks. It is quite uncommon save in the most sun-blessed areas and gives rise to no complaints apart from the obvious cosmetic problems resulting from the odd appearance.

Stellate scars (syn. triradiate scars)

These frequently seen lesions (Figure 2.8) occur predominantly on the dorsa of severely sun-damaged forearms and hands. They are white, irregular angulate scars which often have an overall triradiate or star-shaped configuration. Their owners usually say that the scars are the result of a variety of minor injuries such as knocks and burns, but these attributions are probably rationalizations and in most cases appear to arise spontaneously in an as yet unexplained way. They appear to be permanent and do not give rise to symptoms.

Actinic granuloma

This condition is probably not as uncommon as has been suggested. First described by O'Brien in 1975[6] the condition is characterized clinically by persistent and asymptomatic pink annular lesions and plaques over the forearms and neck. When they are biopsied the histological findings show a characteristic picture of a mixed inflammatory cell infiltrate with some foreign body giant cells surrounding a disorganized relatively acellular area of dermis that does not stain for elastic tissue, although there is considerable elastotic change to either side of the annulus of inflammatory cells. Some have suggested that it may not be a distinct disorder but is a variant of atypical necrobiosis,[7] but the consensus seems to be that it is in fact a separate inflammatory response to the altered dermal connective tissue,[8,9] although we know very little about its pathogenesis. In fact it is not uncommon to find small clusters of inflammatory cells scattered throughout the sun-damaged dermis. Their presence is unexplained.

Raimer's bands

Linear bands composed of flesh-coloured, yellowish papules and plaques have been described affecting the dorsa of the forearms. Such findings seem to be extremely rare as there appears to be only four case reports in the literature.[10] Histologically, there is marked elastotic degenerative change, which has been confirmed in one case by electron microscopy.

Bullous solar elastosis

Looking at histological sections from some patients one feels surprised that bullae do not arise more often. Williams et al[11] describe two patients who did in fact develop blisters on the forearms in areas of skin that were severely sun-damaged. Histologically there was just severe elastosis with irregular clefts and spaces and no other obvious reason for the blistering.

Linear focal elastosis

This condition is characterized by the appearance of horizontal stria-like lines on the back.[12] Histologically there is an increase in the elastic tissue present in the dermis. The cause is unknown, but it does not appear to be due to photodamage and it may even be hamartomatous or perhaps be an odd type of striae distensae.

Solar elastotic degenerative change

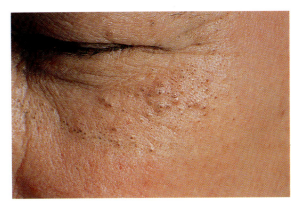

Figure 2.9
Plaque of comedones in intraorbital region of a late middle-aged man.

Senile comedones and sebaceous gland hyperplasia

It is often suggested that senile comedones and senile sebaceous gland hyperplasia are in some way associated with photodamage. Certainly senile comedones do appear to develop at sites of maximum sun damage in some patients—the condition known as the Favre–Racouchot syndrome would appear to be an uncommon but obvious example of this situation. In this degenerative disorder thickened yellowish patches appear on the upper malar regions and at the lateral margins of the orbits studded over which are numerous large

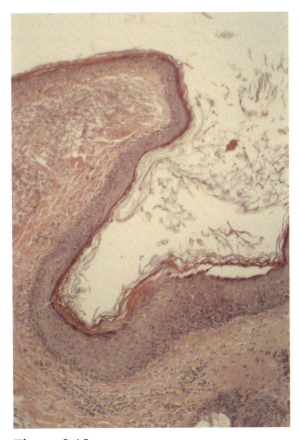
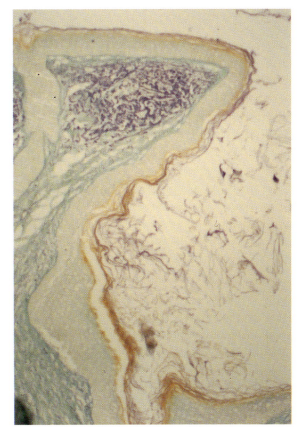

Figure 2.10
Histopathology of dilated follicular cavity from senile comedone. Elastic stain does not reveal a great amount of elastotic change.

comedones (Figure 2.9). Unfortunately, the relationship between these follicular anomalies and solar elastotic degenerative changes does not seem as clear-cut as one might think. When the presence of senile comedones was documented in a residential population of elderly individuals no special correlation was observed with the overall degree of photodamage.[13] Nonetheless, it has to be admitted that in some patients large comedones do develop at sites of maximum sun damage, particularly on the upper cheeks and at the lateral margins of the orbits. It may be that the abnormal dermis of this group of sun-damaged individuals does not provide adequate support for the follicular canal but allows it to dilate in the same way that telangiectasia occurs in blood vessels that are unsupported, which 'fill up' with horny debris. This, however, it must be admitted, does seem somewhat simplistic and there is no real evidence in favour of this concept. In fact, histological examination of senile comedones shows that there is elastosis around the neck of the follicle only and not around the follicular canal (Figure 2.10). Senile comedones are also seen over the nose and elsewhere on the face (Figure 2.11). Giant comedones and other acquired pilosebaceous anomalies certainly occur on the trunk well away from areas of significant photodamage.

In our view sebaceous gland hyperplasia is unlikely to be associated with solar elastotic degeneration other than by chance, although there are several publications suggesting that the stippled appearance over the front of the neck and on the upper chest is due to sebaceous gland hyperplasia in solar elastotic tissue.[14-16] Calderone and Fenske prefer to use the term "striated beaded lines" for this change. In the investigation on senile comedones referred to above, sebaceous gland hyperplasia was also recorded and no association was found between this and the degree of solar elastotic change. It is difficult to believe that the hyperplastic sebaceous gland has been stimulated by solar UVR. Certainly

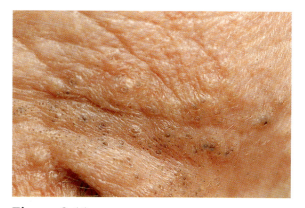

Figure 2.11

Senile comedones over the eyelid in an elderly male.

this odd hyperplastic change may be seen outside sun-exposed areas and its severity seems unrelated to the degree of elastotic change.

Changes to mechanical properties of sun-damaged skin

The mechanical properties of skin affected by solar elastosis are found to be significantly altered compared with normal healthy non-sun-damaged skin in a person of the same age. Pick up a fold of skin from the back of the hand of a photodamaged individual. Now contrast the ease with which this can be done, and the time taken for it to fall back to the level of the skin surface after release, with that of skin from a non-photodamaged matched similarly aged control. It will be evident that photodamaged skin is more lax and less 'springy' (Figures 2.12a, b, c and d).

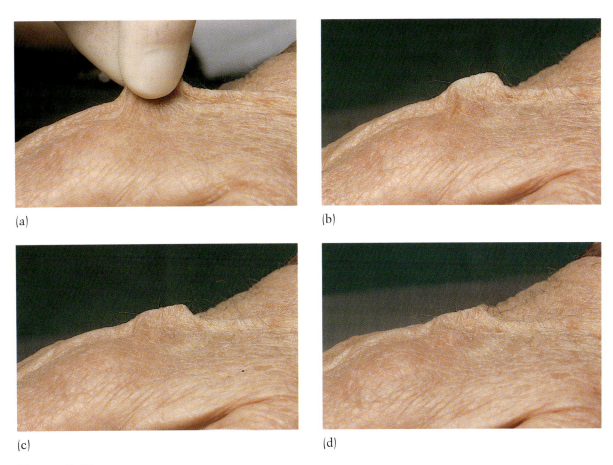

Figure 2.12

(a) A pinch test of skin on back of hand; (b) Immediately after releasing pinch; (c) 5 seconds after releasing pinch; (d) 30 seconds after releasing pinch. It can be seen that the fold of skin persists even up to 30 seconds indicating a loss of the elastic quality of skin.

It should be quite obvious that replacement of normal dermal fibrous connective tissue by a degenerate 'gelatinous' non-fibrous homogeneous material is likely to result in major changes in the way the skin responds to mechanical stresses, but it is quite difficult to characterize and interpret these alterations using the non-invasive instrumentation and techniques available. A quite basic problem is that photodamaged skin is usually the property of individuals who are incidentally chronologically aged anyway and it is impossible to sort out whether the changes recorded are the result of chronic exposure to solar UVR, or due to the processes of intrinsic aging itself, or to both factors. There are also numerous difficulties which are inherent to making this kind of biomechanical measurement in vivo,[17] which include the influence of the orientation in which the measurement is made, the ambient environmental conditions (temperature and humidity in particular) under which the measurement is taken and the recent mechanical stress history of the body part examined. Unfortunately, researchers have also used a motley array of intriguing and innovative instruments with which to interrogate the skin. In addition, they have studied different body sites and employed various experimental conditions, making it impossible to obtain any consistent or coherent view. When one realizes that some of the unexposed sites employed as controls are sometimes not all that unexposed and for the most part there has been little attempt to relate observations to the degree of photodamage sustained, the reasons for there being much confusion in the area become obvious. However, it is true that all studies have been able to demonstrate a reduction in both elasticity and extensibility of significantly photodamaged skin.[18,19] The effects of psoralen plus ultraviolet A (PUVA) therapy on skin have been used as a model for the effects of chronic UVR exposure on the mechanical properties of skin and in both the study by Adhoute et al[20] and that by Barroni et al[21] there was found to be a decrease in both extensibility and in elasticity of affected skin. Our own studies on sun-exposed skin using uniaxial linear extensometry have demonstrated a complex picture with alteration dependent on the orientation of the test and the chronological age of the subject. Overall it was clear that skin elasticity decreased in sun-damaged areas and was stiffer and became much less extensible. In recent years a suction device known as the Cutometer[22] has been employed to characterize the physical properties of skin. It relies on measuring the height of a bubble of skin sucked into a port whose diameter can be changed. Pierard[23] used this instrument with a suction port of 4 mm on the exposed and non-exposed forearm skin of 86 volunteer subjects and noted significant decreases in the maximum deformation on the dorsal exposed surface compared with the ventral surface. These authors also derived a potentially important parameter from their data, which they termed the cutaneous extrinsic aging score (CEAS). This was first derived as follows: CEAS = differential maximum deformation − viscoelastic deformation of skin.

The altered mechanical quality of the abnormal elastotic dermal connective tissue allows the small blood vessels and lymphatics to dilate because of the decrease in perivascular supporting dermal connective tissue. The lack of investing collagen fibres also makes the thin-walled blood vessels vulnerable to external mechanical traumata so that quite large ecchymoses often develop in severely sun-damaged sites. These purple patches, which are inappropriately known as 'senile purpura' but would be better described as 'solar purpura', are usually 0.5–2.0 cm^2 in size but may be larger. Although technically bruises they are much more persistent and may take some weeks before finally disappearing. Presumably deficient macrophage activity in the elderly and disturbed tissue architecture in sun-damaged skin contributes to the persistence of these lesions.[24]

Clearly, the older one becomes, the more solar damage will accumulate in the sun-exposed dermis, but apart from this relationship alterations in the dermal connective tissue due to the aging process sui generis are quite unlike those due to solar elastosis. In intrinsic aging the dermal collagen becomes more insoluble and the collagen molecules develop more cross-links with the passing of the years.[25] At the same time the weight of collagen per unit skin surface area drops as a function of age[26] and the interfibrillary proteoglycan ground substance decreases. The net result of these alterations is that the skin becomes thinner and stiffer (see also Chapter 5). There have been at least two studies using pulsed A-scan ultrasound techniques that have demonstrated that there is a significant reduction in skin thickness with increasing age.[27,28] There is about a 30 per cent reduction in dermal thickness between the ages of 20 and 80, although most of thinning seems to take place after the age of 50. Solar

Solar elastotic degenerative change

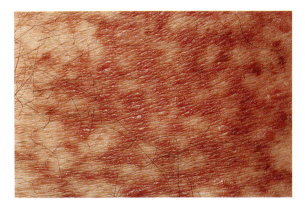

Figure 2.13
Erythema ab igne due to persistent heating of skin of legs.

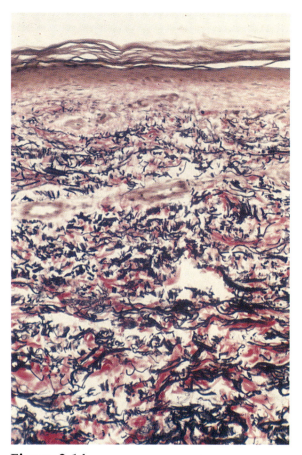

Figure 2.14
Patch of erythema ab igne. Elastic stain to show excess elastic tissue throughout dermis.

elastosis first becomes evident histologically in the fair-skinned inhabitant of sunny countries when he or she is in their early twenties and clinically the characteristic fine lines and subtle colour changes begin just a little later in the late twenties or early thirties. A dark skin does not completely protect against photodamage—this depends on the total dose of UVR received and possibly the dose rate.

The pathology of solar elastosis

The dermal changes of solar elastosis are both quantitative and qualitative. The term 'elastosis' (or elastotic degeneration) refers to the finding that the normal dermal fibrous connective tissue is replaced in sun-exposed sites by an abnormal substance that stains for elastic tissue when elastic tissue stains such as elastica van Gieson or Halmi's stain are used. The sites involved are those that are usually directly exposed to the sun, i.e. the face and neck, the dorsa of the hands and the dorsal aspects of the forearms. Other sites such as the bald scalp and the front of the chest may also be affected, depending on the prevailing customs and clothing fashions. Other areas occasionally develop elastotic degenerative change dependent on the same two factors—for example the skin of the lower legs in women—especially if the condition known as erythema ab igne is present. In this disorder skin persistently exposed to focal sources of heat become damaged and develops a brown reticulate pattern (Figure 2.13). The elastotic change observed in erythema ab igne is similar to that caused by the sun, but extends deeper into the dermis (Figure 2.14),

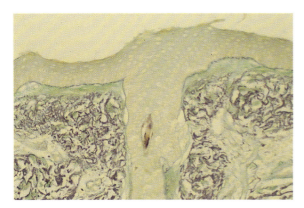

Figure 2.15

Patch of photodamaged skin stained to show elastic tissue in the sub epidermal zone. Note that there is an area immediately beneath the epidermis uninvolved by the elastotic change. This is known as the grenz zone.

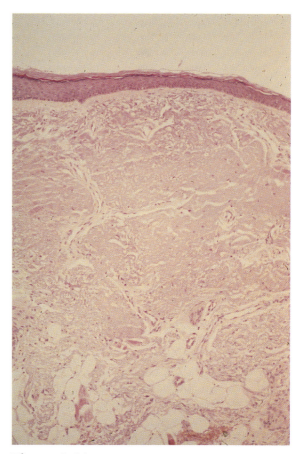

Figure 2.16

Histopathology of photodamaged area to show loss of fibrillar component of dermis and homogenization of connective tissue. (haemotoxylin–eosin ×15).

presumably because infrared irradiation penetrates more deeply into the skin UVR.

Interestingly, the dermal abnormality seems always to start at the same point vertically within the skin. It begins at the point some 20–50 μm beneath the epidermis—the uninvolved dermal band immediately subjacent to the epidermis being known as the grenz zone (Figure 2.15). Lavker[29] has likened this Grenz zone to a healing wound, as reticulin is found here indicating new connective tissue synthesis. The vertical depth within the skin that is reached by the elastotic material is roughly proportional to the total accumulated UVR dose. The same applies to the density of the elastotic tissue per unit area and the proportion of the horizontal length of the skin occupied by the abnormal material.

The morphology of the elastotic material within the dermis is somewhat variable but the loss of the normal fibrillary pattern to the collagenous dermis is the prime structural change observed. The appearance of homogeneous blobs of elastotic staining material is an important characteristic of the abnormal dermal connective tissue (Figure 2.16).

Another less frequent appearance of the abnormal elastotic dermis is of broad irregularly arranged bands of short length which can be described as chopped up 'spaghetti'. Because the homogenous material is sometimes broken up into rounded globular masses it does not tax the imagination overmuch to describe the appearance as 'spaghetti and meatball like' when the globular masses of elastotic material occur together with the tangled broken bands (Figure 2.17).

Solar elastotic degenerative change

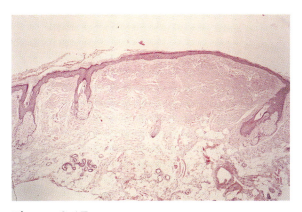

Figure 2.17
Histopathology of photodamaged area to show a mixture of homogenized zones and fibrillar components giving rise to spaghetti and meatball appearance (haemotoxylin–eosin ×10).

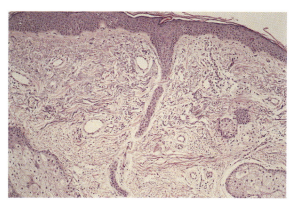

Figure 2.18
There are many telangiectetic vessels in the upper dermis in this histological section with thickened capillary walls (haemotoxylin–eosin ×30).

The blood vessels set in this deformed and disorganized dermis are decreased in number and are markedly and irregularly dilated, accounting for the telangiectasia observed clinically. The vascular dilation seems to be due to the disappearance of the normal supporting perivascular collagenous connective tissue, but there appears to be a reduction in papillary capillaries and the small vessels themselves are also slightly thickened. The dilated small blood vessels in many instances also show thickening of their walls (Figure 2.18) and ultrastructurally an 'onion ring' arrangement of fibres is observed around some of the vessels.[30]

One somewhat unexpected and interesting finding in solar elastosis is the presence of mixed inflammatory cell infiltrate that is usually present to a variable extent. This cellular infiltrate appears early on in the process and contains degranulating mast cells.[31] There is a mixture of lymphocytes, macrophages and mast cells scattered throughout the elastotic material. Although the inflammatory cells do not appear to have any special anatomical arrangement there is a tendency for the cellular infiltrate to be perivascular.[32] Whether the foci of granulomatous inflammation containing giant cells and epithelioid cells, which are found in elastotic skin encircling non-elastotic areas and known as actinic granulomata, are an extension of the more frequently seen inflammation referred to above is unknown. The granulomas are of variable size and shape and as yet there is no adequate explanation for their presence (Figure 2.19).

It has been suggested that the cellular inflammation observed in sun-damaged areas and described above is in fact a fundamental component of the elastotic degeneration and may be important in the pathogenesis of solar elastotic degenerative change.

Routine staining of tissue sections with haematoxylin and eosin demonstrates that the abnormal dermis is distinctly more basophilic then the normal dermis and that it is patchily positive for proteoglycan when tested for with periodic acid Schiff reagent, alcian blue or Hale stain. The most dramatic feature is the strong staining for elastic tissue with all the usual elastic stains, including the

24 Photodamaged Skin: Clinical Signs, Causes and Management

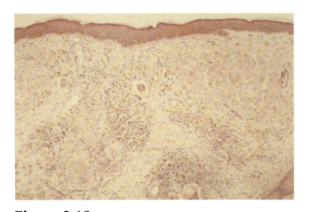

Figure 2.19
Pathology of actinic granuloma showing areas of granulomatous inflammation (×30).

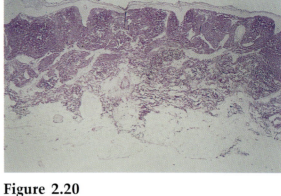

Figure 2.20
Photomicrograph of section of photodamaged skin stained with elastic tissue to show dense elastic staining in the upper and mid dermis.

orcein-based reagents such as Verhoeff's stain and van Gieson's stain or others such as Halmi's stain (Figure 2.20). Ultrastructurally, evidence of elastogenesis is an early change, but later on masses of irregularly arranged elastic tissue may be observed containing variable amounts of disorganized microfibrillar and electron dense homogenous components[33] (Figure 2.21). In addition, microfibres with a long internal cross-banding pattern are seen which are known as 'zebra fibres'[34]—their significance is not clear.

The pathogenesis of solar elastosis

Our knowledge of the pathogenesis of solar elastosis is incomplete. At one time it was even uncertain whether the elastic staining material found in solar elastosis was in fact genuine elastic tissue. This at least now seems certain from work by the Uitto group[35,36] and others[37,38] which has established that the abnormal material is essentially elastin biochemically, although disorganized and abnormal in the proportions of its various constituents. There is much less agreement as to how and why the elastotic material accumulates. There are several different possible mechanisms and they are not necessarily mutually incompatible. A once popular hypothesis was that solar UVR caused the transformation of normal dermal collagen into the degenerate elastic-staining substance seen in sun-damaged skin. This would not explain the subepidermal uninvolved grenz zone or the apparent absence of intermediate forms of connective tissue morphologically. A similar and somewhat more plausible suggestion is that the abnormal elastotic material derives from the pre-existing normal elastic network. Pravata et al[39], employing the N-(7-dimethylamino-4 methyl-3 coumarinyl maleimide) (DACM) fluorescence technique to detect S–S and -SH bonds in sun-damaged and control skin, found heavy fluorescence for S-S bands in dense elastotic masses. Fluorescence for -S–S and -SH bonds were present in less-damaged areas and they suggested that solar elastosis could be the consequence of a defect in degradation or synthesis of elastic fibres.

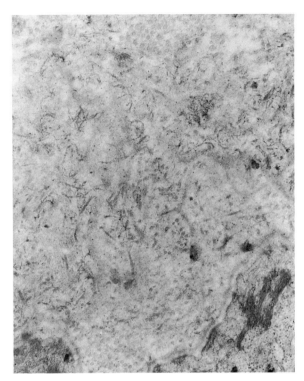

Figure 2.21
Electron micrograph of biopsy from photodamaged skin on forearm showing extensive elastotic degenerative change. There are many small irregularly arranged microfibrils and clumps of homogenous material.

Lysozyme has been found in excessive amounts in sun-damaged dermis[40] and its presence may indicate another way in which the elastotic material may accumulate. Lysozyme is a protein that inhibits elastase and collagenase and may allow a build up of abnormal quantities of elastotic material.

As UVB, a substantial proportion of solar UVR, does not penetrate much further into the skin than the basal layer of the epidermis it has seemed reasonable to suggest that the initiating stimulus to the development of solar elastosis is in fact to the epidermis. It has been shown that after UVR damage to epidermal keratinocytes, cytokines such as tumour necrosis factor-α are released that can influence the synthetic activities of fibroblasts.[41,42] This sequence of events might also explain the accumulation of inflammatory cells in sun-damaged skin, since accompanying or following the release of cytokines, adhesion molecules are released attracting inflammatory cells into the area. Some have put forward the idea that the presence of inflammation is a fundamental component of solar elastosis and responsible for the elastotic degenerative change rather than being secondary to it. Increased collagenase activity has been detected in solar elastosis,[43] but it is difficult to see how this could be the primary abnormality resulting in the connective tissue change. Whatever the primary metabolic injury there seems little doubt that there is increased synthesis of elastic tissue, as the Uitto group have shown increased levels of RNA for elastin and fibrillin in areas of solar elastotic degenerative change.[44] This group have performed some very elegant studies with transgenic mice in which the elastin promotor gene has been linked to a chloramphenicol acetyl transferase reporter gene. When such mice are irradiated with UVB, elastic tissue accumulates. UVA irradiation also increased elastin but was very much less potent than UVB.

Other interesting observations concerning the pathogenesis of elastosis include those of the Ann Arbor group who have demonstrated firstly increased collagenase (and other metalloproteinases such as stromolysin and gelatinase) activities after acute UVR injury.[45] They have also detected decreases in collagen precursors procollagens I and III in chronically photodamaged skin which correlate with the degree of photodamage.[46]

Models for solar elastosis

Models for solar elastosis are needed for two major purposes. Without a model it is difficult to investigate the different hypotheses which attempt to explain the development of the disorder. The other major use of a model system is to screen and test agents of potential use in the treatment or prevention or solar elastosis.

The development of elastotic degenerative change in the dermis of the skin of hairless mice after irradiation by UVB as described by L Kligman seems currently the best system available.[47] Kligman and Sayre investigated the action spectrum for solar elastosis in this model employing an image analytical method to measure the degree of elastosis induced.[48] The mouse model has also been used to detect and measure the broadening of the subepidermal repair zone in the skin of mice with elastotic changes after use of topical tretinoin[49] and topical isotretinoin.[50] Similarly, it has been used to show that topical tretinoin will reduce the atrophogenic effect of potent topical corticosteroids without interfering with the anti-inflammatory effect of the steroid on the skin.

A development of this mouse model has been described by Uitto's group in Philadelphia. They have used a transgenic mouse line 'that expresses' the human elastin promoter/chloramphenicol aminotransferase (CAT) construct in a tissue-specific and developmentally regulated manner. They have used this model to investigate the action spectrum of solar elastosis and found that although UVA had some activity in stimulating elastosis, UVB was by far the most effective waveband. They have also employed the transgenic model to look at the efficacy of sunscreens in preventing elastosis.

The ideal model of solar elastotic change would be in man. In such a model it may be possible to induce solar elastosis in small areas of normally non-exposed skin of human volunteer subjects. The longest period over which we have repeatedly irradiated the skin of volunteer subjects with UVR has been 4 weeks, though we have employed a regimen of irradiation with infrared over a 6-week period to study the effects of heating. It seems intrinsically unlikely that any relevant changes in dermal connective tissue would be induced by experimental irradiation for periods of less than 3 or 4 months. It is, however, more than possible that an early marker of solar elastotic change will be identified long before the gross morphological alterations occur. Experimental work in this area continues and it seems likely that a human in vivo model for solar elastosis will develop in the not too distant future.

In vitro 'models' have been employed to investigate the effects of UVR on fibroblasts and the effects of cytokines released after UVR stimulus on fibroblasts and the effects of cytokines release after a UVR stimulus on fibroblast synthetic activity.[51,52] The results of such studies are interesting, but it is difficult to know how relevant they are to the genesis of solar elastosis in vivo.

Treatment of solar elastosis

This subject is dealt with extensively in Chapter 8. There is a tendency for a 'spontaneous improvement' or healing to take place, although the extent to which this can occur is uncertain and anyway depends on stopping any further sun damage. Recent studies suggest that use of sunscreens alone do produce a reduction in the amount of solar damage present.[53]

References

1. Benedetto AV, The environment and skin aging. *Clinics in Derm* (1998) **16**: 129–39.
2. Long CC, Marks R, Increased risk of skin cancer: Another Celtic Myth? *J Am Acad Dermatol* (1995) **33**: 659–61.

3. Warren R, Garstein V, Kligman AM et al, Age, sunlight and facial skin: A histologic and quantative study. *J Am Acad Dermatol* (1991) **25**: 751–60.
4. Daniels HW, Smoker's wrinkles. *Ann Intern Med* (1971) **75**: 873–80.
5. Marks R, Harcourt-Webster JN, The histopathology of rosacea. *Arch Dermatol* (1969) **100**: 683–92.
6. O'Brien JP, Actinic granuloma, an annular connective tissue disorder affecting sun and heat damaged (elastotic) skin. *Arch Dermatol* (1975) **111**: 460–66.
7. Ragaz Z, Ackerman AB, Is actinic granuloma a specific condition? *Am J Dermatopath* (1979) **1**: 43–50.
8. McGrae JD, Actinic granuloma: a clinical, histopathologic and immunocytochemical study. *Arch Dermatol* (1986) **122**: 43–7.
9. Hanke CW, Bailin PL, Roenigk HH Jr, Annular elastolytic giant cell granuloma. *J Am Acad Dermatol* (1979) **1**: 413–21.
10. Raimer SS, Sanchez RL, Hubler WR Jr et al, Solar elastotic bands of the forearm: an unusual clinical presentation of actinic elastosis. *J Am Acad Dermatol* (1986) **15**: 650–6.
11. Williams BT, Barr RJ, Dutta B, Bullous solar elastosis. *J Am Acad Dermatol* (1996) **34**: 856–8.
12. Fenske NA, Lober CW, Aging and its effects on the skin. In: SL Moschella, HJ Hurley (eds) *Dermatology*. WB Saunders: Philadelphia, 1992, pp. 107–22.
13. Kumar R, Marks R, Sebaceous gland hyperplasia and senile comedones: a prevalence study in elderly hospitalised patients. *Br J Dermatol* (1987) **117**: 231–6.
14. Even Paz Z, Sagher I, Cutis punctate linearis colli: stippled skin. *Dermatologica* (1963) **126**: 1–12.
15. Fenske NA, Lober CW, Aging and its effects on the skin. In: SL Moschella, HJ Hurley (eds) *Dermatology*. WB Saunders: Philadelphia, 1992, pp. 107–22.
16. Calderone CD, Fenske NA, The clinical spectrum of actinic elastosis. *J Am Acad Dermatol* (1995) **32**: 1016–24.
17. Marks R, Edwards C, Mechanical properties of the dermis: an engineer's nightmare. In: CM Lapiére, T Krieg (eds) *Connective Tissue Diseases of the Skin*. Marcel Dekker: New York, 1993, pp. 103–16.
18. Pierard GE, Kort R, Letawe C et al, Biomechanical assessment of photodamage. Derivation of a cutaneous extrinsic aging score. *Skin Res Tech* (1995) **1**: 17–20.
19. Leveque JL, Porte G, De Rigal et al, Influence of chronic sun exposure on some biophysical parameters of the human skin: an in vivo study. *J Cut Aging Cosmetic Derm* (1998/9) **1**: 123–7.
20. Adhoute H, Rigal J, Marchand JP et al, Influence of age and sun exposure on the biophysical properties of the human skin: an in vivo study. *Photoderm, Photoimmunol Photomed* (1992) **9**: 99–103.
21. Borroni G, Zaccone C, Vignati G et al, Assessment of biomechanical changes induced by long term PUVA treatment (> 1000 J/sqcm) in psoriatic patients (abstract). 8th International Symposium on Bioengineering and the Skin. Stresa, Italy, June 1990: 59.
22. Couturaud V, Coutable J, Kaiat A, Skin biomechanical properties: in vivo evaluation of influence of age and body site by a non invasive method. *Skin Res Tech* (1995) **1**: 68–73.
23. Piérard GE, Kort R, Letawe C et al, Biomechanical assessment of photodamage: Derivation of a cutaneous extrinsic aging score. *Skin Res Tech* (1995) **1**: 17–20.
24. Shuster S, Scarborough H, Senile purpura. *Quart J Med* (1961) **30**: 33–40.
25. Hall DA, *The Aging of Connective Tissue*. Academic Press: London, 1976.
26. Shuster S, Black MM, McVitie E, The influence of age and sex on skin thickness, skin collagen and density. *Br J Dermatol* (1975) **93**: 639–43.
27. Tan CY, Statham B, Marks R et al, Skin thickness measurement by pulsed ultrasound: its reproducibility, validation and variability. *Br J Dermatol* (1982) **106**: 657–67.
28. Escoffier C, de Rigal J, Rochefort A et al, Age related mechanical properties of human skin: An in vivo study. *J Invest Dermatol* (1989) **93**: 353–7.
29. Lavker RM, Cutaneous aging: Chronological versus photoaging. In: BA Gilchrest (ed.) *Photoaging*. Blackwell Science: Cambridge, MA, 1995, pp. 123–35.
30. Motley RJ, Barton SP, Marks R, The significance of telengiectasia in rosacea. In: R Marks, G Plewig (eds) *Acne and Related Disorders*. Martin Dunitz: London, 1989, pp. 339–44.

31. Lavker RM, Kligman AM, Chronic heliodermatitis: a morphological evaluation of chronic actinic dermal damage with emphasis on the role of mast cells. *J Invest Dermatol* (1988) **90**: 325–30.
32. Labker RM, Structural alterations in exposed and unexposed aged skin. *J Invest Dermatol* (1979) **73**: 59–66.
33. Stevanovic DV, Elastotic degeneration. A light and electron microscopic study. *Br J Dermatol* (1976) **94**: 23.
34. Zheng P, Kligman LH, UVA induced ultrastructural changes in hairless mouse skin: A comparison to UVB induced damage. *J Invest Dermatol* (1993) **100**: 194–9.
35. Bernstein EF, Chen YQ, Kopp JB et al, Long term sun exposure alters the collagen of the papillary dermis. *J Am Acad Dermatol* (1996) **34**: 209–18.
36. Bernstein EF, Brown DB, Urbach F et al, Ultraviolet radiation activated the human elastin promoter in transgenic mice: A novel in vivo and in vitro model of cutaneous photoaging. *J Invest Dermatol* (1995) **105**: 269–73.
37. Lovell C, Plastow SR, Russell-Jones R et al, Collagen and elastin in actinic elastosis. *J Invest Dermatol* (1984) **82**: 566.
38. Chen V, Fleischmajer R, Schwartz E et al, Immunochemistry of elastotic material in sun damaged skin. *J Invest Dermatol* (1986) **87**: 334–7.
39. Pravata G, Noto G, Amco M, Increased SS bonds in chronic solar elastosis: a study with N-(7-dimethylamino-4-methyl-3-coumarinyl) molamide (DACM) stain. *J Derm Sci* (1994) **7**: 14–23.
40. Albrecht S, From L, Kahn HJ, Lysosyme in abnormal dermal elastic fibers of cutaneous aging, solar elastosis and pseudoxanthoma elasticum. *J Cut Path* (1991) **18**: 75–81.
41. Scharffetter-Kochanek K, Wlaschek M, Bolsen K, Herrmann G et al, Mechanisms of cutaneous photoaging. In: R Marks, G Plewig (eds) *The Environmental Threat to the Skin*. Martin Dunitz: London, 1989, pp. 77–82.
42. Oxholm A, Oxholm P, Staberg B et al, Immunohistological detection of interleukin I-like molecules and tumor necrosis factor in human epidermis before and after UVB irradiation in vivo. *Br J Dermatol* (1988) **118**: 493–503.
43. Schwartz E, Cruickshank FA, Christensen CC et al, Collagen alterations in chronically sun damaged human skin. *Photochem Photobiol* (1993) **58**: 841–4.
44. Berstein EF, Chen YQ, Tamai K et al, Enhanced elastin and fibrillin gene expression in chronically photodamaged skin. *J Invest Dermatol* (1994) **103**: 182–6.
45. Fisher GJ, Wang Z, Datta SC et al, Pathophysiology of premature skin aging induced by ultaviolet light. *N Engl J Med* (1997) **337**: 1419–28.
46. Talwar HS, Griffiths CEM, Fisher GJ et al, Reduced type I and type II procollagens in photodamaged adult human skin. *J Invest Dermatol* (1995) **105**: 285–90.
47. Kligman LH, Animal models of photodamage and its treatment. In: BA Gilchrest (ed.) *Photodamage*. Blackwell Science: Cambridge, MA, 1995, pp. 136–56.
48. Kligman LH, Sayre RM, An action spectrum for ultraviolet induced elastosis in hairless mice. Quantification of elastosis by image analysis. *Photochem Photobiol* (1991) **53**: 237–42.
49. Kligman LH, Effects of all-trans etinoic acid on the dermis of hairless mice. *J Am Acad Dermatol* (1986) **15**: 779–85.
50. Bernstein EF, Brown DB, Takeuchi T et al, Evaluation of sunscreens with various sun protection factors in a new transgenic mouse model of cutaneous photoaging that measures elastin promotor activation. *J Am Acad Dermatol* (1997) **37**: 725–9.
51. Kossodo S de, Cruz PD Jr, Dougherty I et al, Expression of the tumor necrosis factor gene by dermal fibroblasts in response to ultraviolet irradiation or lipopolysaccharide. *J Invest Dermatol* (1995) **104**: 318–22.
52. Werth VP, Williams KJ, Fisher EA et al, UVB irradiation alters cellular responses to cytokines: role in extracellular matrix gene expression. *J Invest Dermatol* (1997) **108**: 290–4.
53. Boyd AS, Naylor M, Camcron GS ct al, The effects of chronic sunscreen use on the histologic changes of dermatoheliosis. *J Am Acad Dermatol* (1995) **33**: 941–6.

3 Dyspigmentation and melanoma

Introduction

Ultraviolet (UV) irradiation-induced damage to the skin induces a cascade of cellular and molecular events involving all cell types, including melanocytes. Acute exposure to UV induces tanning, with two types of photobiological reaction of the melanin pigmentary system forming the basis of this phenomenon: the immediate pigment-darkening reaction; and delayed tanning, which is considered to be a photoprotective mechanism of the skin. Repeated exposure to UV radiation particularly to sunlight, induces cumulative skin changes which vary considerably in severity between individuals, undoubtedly reflecting inherent differences in vulnerability to solar insult and the ability to repair.

The clinical features of actinically damaged skin are somewhat different from those due to chronological aging. In the epidermis, melanin pigment is a good indicator of the photodamage and pigmentary changes are one of the most visible markers of photoaged skin.[1] Exposed skin in the elderly is usually unevenly pigmented with a mottled appearance, demonstrating that chronic exposure to UV radiation plays role in the induction of these modifications, and may severely damage the melanocyte system of the skin, resulting in both hyper- and hypomelanotic lesions.

Clinical description

Hypermelanotic lesions

Mottling

Photoaged skin is often characterized by mottled, irregular areas of pigmentation (Figure 3.1), which is paradoxical as the number of epidermal melanocytes in aged skin is decreased compared with the number in young adult skin. This clinical appearance is probably explained by the increased dopa-positivity of melanocytes in the chronically sun-exposed skin and by an irregular distribution of

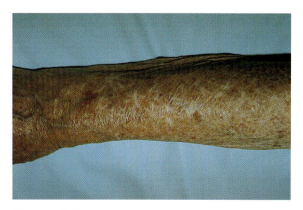

Figure 3.1

Mottling of photodamaged skin.

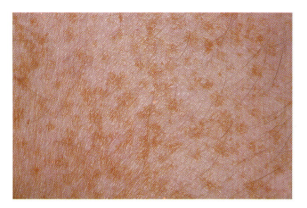

Figure 3.2
Multiple ephelides.

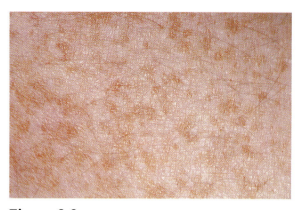

Figure 3.3
Ephelides: high-power view.

the pigment cells, as well as by an irregular distribution of melanosomes within epidermal keratinocytes.

Light microscopy of photodamaged skin demonstrates melanocyte hypertrophy and hyperplasia associated with an heterogeneous distribution of melanin granules. The distribution of melanocytes along the basal layer is irregular, this probably accounting for the characteristic mottled appearance of chronically sun-exposed aged skin. By electron microscopy, it can be seen that there is a considerable heterogeneity of morphological and functional characteristics of melanocytes.[2] Most of them are very large, showing changes indicative of hyperstimulation, but others have ceased melanogenesis. They contain only few fully melanized melanosomes; they have little cytoplasm while in some areas there are no dendrites.

Ephelides

These small brown macules or freckles (a few millimetres in diameter) (Figures 3.2 and 3.3) may be considered to be a sign of photoaging in genetically predisposed individuals. Previous genetic studies suggest that freckling is determined by an autosomal dominant gene. However, the hypothesis that this feature is due to somatic mutations of epidermal melanocytes induced by ultraviolet irradiation (UVR) has also been raised. Ephelides appear in childhood and increase in number in adults. They are always multiple, scattered over sun-exposed skin (most commonly the nose, cheeks, shoulders and extensor aspects of the arms), and become darker after exposure to sun. Clinical evidence indicates that fair skin, red or light hair colour, light eye colour and freckles are phenotypic markers of increased susceptibility to sun-induced skin damage. The presence of freckles is associated with a 2.5-fold increase in the rate of sunburn susceptibility and poor tanning compared with individuals without this feature. The contribution of freckling to a lower minimal erythemal dose (MED) is skin-type-dependent. It increases the likelihood of a lower MED value in individuals with skin types I and II 2.9-fold, compared with non-freckled persons with skin type III, while in skin type III it decreases this risk by 0.4.[3]

When examined using light microscopy, ephelides are characterized by hyperpigmentation of the epidermal basal cell layer, without elongation of the rete ridges. On split skin preparations stained by the dopa reaction, freckled skin has significantly fewer melanocytes per square millimetre than adjacent paler skin, but the melanocytes are larger and are strongly dopa-positive. Electron microscopic studies show that the melanocytes in freckles produce large numbers of mature melanosomes similar to those seen in dark-skinned individuals (rod-like shape with a striated internal structure), but they are different from those of adjacent paler skin (round with a granular internal structure). These observations led to the suggestion that the epidermis of freckled individuals contains two types of melanocytes with different capacities for melanogenesis. In the light of the recent advances in the understanding of melanogenesis and its genetic control, it may be suggested that melanosomes in freckled human epidermis are eumelanosomes, i.e. melanosomes associated with dark eumelanin production, and melanosomes in paler skin adjacent to freckles are phaeomelanosomes, i.e. associated with reddish-yellow phaeomelanin. Eumelanin is photoprotective whereas phaeomelanin, because of its potential to generate free radicals in response to UVR, may contribute to UV-induced skin damage. In mammals, the relative proportions of phaeomelanin and eumelanin are regulated by melanocyte-stimulating hormone (MSH), which acts via a receptor on melanocytes to increase the synthesis of eumelanins. Recent genetic findings suggest that the same mechanisms occur in humans. Indeed, sequence variants of the melanocyte-stimulating hormone receptor gene MC1R are associated with red hair, fair skin and freckling in humans,[4] that is, a 'phaeomelanotic phenotype'. This suggests that the MSH receptor gene is involved either directly or indirectly in the genetic control of freckling.

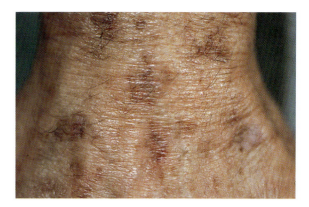

Figure 3.4

Actinic lentigo: typical distribution on the dorsum of hands and wrists.

Actinic lentigo (senile lentigo)

This condition, also known as solar lentigo, commonly occurs as multiple lesions in areas of skin chronically exposed to the sun. These lentigines, which are benign, hyperpigmented macules, varying in size from a few millimetres to more than 1 cm across, may coalesce and their borders may be regular or irregular (Figures 3.4–3.6). Great variations in the shape have been observed and they are usually dark brown, although yellow, light brown or even black lesions are not uncommon. A mottled appearance, due to varying degrees of hyperpigmentation, may occur within lesions. There is no scaling, desquamation, hyperkeratosis or infiltration. Solar lentigines darken significantly after exposure to sunlight, even at infraerythemal doses. Chromometric quantification of these pigmentary changes demonstrates an increase in the red and yellow colour components. The incidence of actinic lentigo increases with age: 25–50 per cent of people over the age of 50 years and 90 per cent of subjects between 80 and 100 years age have actinic lentigines. Their incidence is about the same in both sexes and they are equally common in persons of light and dark complexion. The presence of actinic

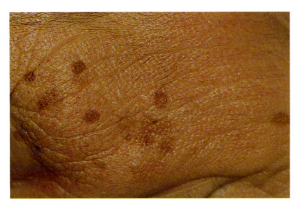

Figure 3.5

Actinic lentigo: tiny pigmented macules of the forehead.

Figure 3.6

Actinic lentigo: note the great variations in the shape and size of the lesions.

lentigines is related to a tendency to freckling in adolescence (relative risk = 2.0) and to two or more episodes of sunburn after the age of 20 (relative risk = 1.6).[5]

The most prominent histological features include hyperpigmentation of the basal cell layer with a marked increase in the number of epidermal dopa-positive melanocytes and elongation of the rete ridges, which appear either club-shaped or tortuous with bud-like extensions. When examined using electron microscopy, epidermal melanocytes display increased activity, with nuclei being irregularly shaped and their cytoplasm containing large numbers of melanosomes. There is no pleomorphism of melanosomes and no atypical cytological alterations of melanocytes.[6] The keratinocytes contain increased numbers of melanosomes and melanosome complexes, and melanosomes are also seen in the horny layer, suggesting that in addition to the increase in the number of melanocytes and increased melanin synthesis there is also an abnormality in the lysosomal degradation of pigment granules within the epidermal keratinocytes.

Actinic lentigo may be extremely difficult to distinguish from the other pigmented lesions present on the skin of almost all elderly patients, including pigmented actinic keratosis, flat pigmented seborrhoeic keratoses, ephelides and naevocellular naevi. However, they are the commonest pigmented lesions on the exposed areas of this age group. The actinic lentigo may rarely present as a black irregular macule, suggesting melanoma. This unusual variant of actinic lentigo is distinct clinically because of its small size (1.5–5 mm), its very dark pigmentation and beaded irregular outline. It has a reticulated pattern and most resembles a spot of ink on the skin. This lesion is found in fair-skinned individuals and in sun-exposed areas of the body, as is classic actinic lentigo. However, the large number of actinic lentigines is in contrast with the presence of only one or a few (≤ 4) 'ink spot' lentigines.[7] Because of its clinical features, this lesion has been named 'reticulated black solar lentigo'. Clinically, skip areas may be seen in the central as well as at the peripheral portions of the lesion.[7] Histologically, these ink spot lentigines show lentiginous hyperplasia with elongation of the rete ridges, marked hyperpigmentation of the epidermal basal layer skip without pigment, involving the suprapapillary

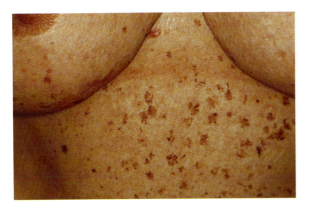

Figure 3.7
Multiple UVA lentigines on the anterior trunk of a 42-year-old woman.

Figure 3.8
UVA lentigo: note the irregular borders of the lesions and their typical stellate appearance.

epidermis and/or the rete ridges. The number of intraepidermal dopa-reactive melanocytes in black lentigines is not significantly different from that in the adjacent normal skin. However, the dendrites of the lesional melanocytes are thicker and more prominent. Occasional hypertrophic melanocytes may be seen. Ultrastructural observations demonstrate an increased number of single or complexed melanosomes in the cytoplasm of keratinocytes. The clinical and histological features of reticulated black solar lentigo are typical and suggest a clinical diagnosis of a benign pigmented lesion.

UVA and PUVA lentigines

UVA lentigines. Several case reports have suggested that UVA alone or UVA contaminated by small amounts of UVB may induce melanocytic lesions, and with the increasing use of sunbeds throughout the year to promote tanning, this problem will probably become more common.[8] Subjects with fair skin who are chronically exposing themselves to UV radiation by using sunbeds should be aware of this potential side-effect since they appear to be most at risk. UVA-lentigines, which develop in areas exposed to radiation, are variable in size and are unevenly pigmented with irregular borders (Figures 3.7 and 3.8); sometimes they have a stellate appearance. Histological examination of the lesions has demonstrated increased numbers of large melanocytes in the epidermal layer with some of these cells showing cellular atypia.[9] Ultrastructural examination has revealed features similar to other forms of lentigo, with melanosome complexes within melanocytes and keratinocytes containing large numbers of melanosomes (Figures 3.9 and 3.10).

UVA lentigines can occur in subjects who have not been using psoralens either topically or orally at the time of UVA irradiation, demonstrating that UVA alone can induce melanocytic lesions resembling those observed in some patients receiving long-term photochemotherapy (see below); both acute and chronic overexposure can apparently induce 'sunbed lentigines'. The long-term behaviour of UVA lentigines is unknown, but the occurrence of melanocytic atypia and melanosomal pleomorphism

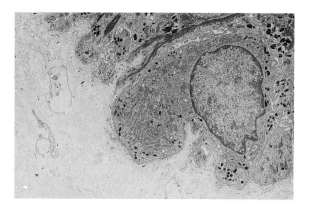

Figure 3.9

UVA lentigo (electron microscopy): a large melanocyte bulging in the underlying dermis is loaded with melanosomes.

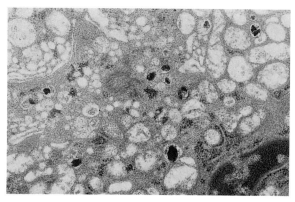

Figure 3.10

UVA lentigo (electron microscopy): typical melanosome pleomorphism.

suggests that all patients should be carefully followed up.

PUVA lentigines. The formation of lentigines in a common side-effect of chronic oral psoralen photochemotherapy.[10] These lesions, known as PUVA lentigines, which appear after 2–3 years of extensive treatment with PUVA, are clinically slightly different from senile lentigines. They are usually smaller, more numerous and more densely scattered than solar lentigines and can be observed in all PUVA-treated areas but occur most frequently on the thighs, groin, buttocks, flanks and arms. The most prominent feature of PUVA lentigines is histological elongation of rete ridges with proliferation of functionally active melanocytes. Other features are dyskeratotic cells, enlarged nuclei in keratinocytes and giant keratinocytes. In contrast to solar lentigines, the melanocytes have highly irregular nuclear contours, occasional prominent nuclei and dendrites that are more numerous and longer.[6] Melanosome alterations are common, including melanosomal pleomorphism and melanin macroglobules.[6]

The mechanism of development of PUVA lentigines is unknown and it has not been established whether the melanocyte and keratinocyte abnormalities observed are a reversible effect of PUVA therapy or whether these lesions are potentially malignant. A precise follow-up of patients with PUVA lentigines is strongly recommended.

Pigmented actinic keratoses and spreading pigmented actinic keratosis

Actinic keratosis (AK) is a premalignant epidermal tumour of sun-exposed skin that can rarely eventually evolve into squamous cell carcinoma of the skin. AKs are usually less than 1 cm in diameter. Their surface is smooth, but may be scaly or verrucous on an erythematous background (Figure 3.11). The classic AK is thought of as a non-pigmented lesion, but pigmented forms may also occur. These pigmented AKs are probably much more common that the literature would indicate.

Clinically, brownish pigmented lesions on sun-exposed skin, similar to lentigo simplex, actinic lentigo, pigmented seborrhoeic keratoses and lentigo, with microscopic

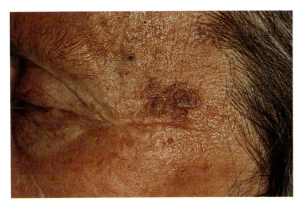

Figure 3.11
Pigmented actinic keratosis. Clinically it is extremely difficult to differentiate this lesion from flat pigmented seborrhoeic keratosis or actinic lentigo.

features of solar keratoses are common. Histologically, these lesions show varying degrees of hyperkeratosis, spotty parakeratosis, acanthosis and finger-like projections and budding of atypical keratinocytes in the lower epidermis, all features typical of AK. In addition, there is an increased amount of melanization in the epidermal basal layer, and numerous melanophages in the upper dermis. The epidermal melanocyte number is not increased and the pigment cells have a normal morphology. Interestingly, there is no increase in the amount of melanin pigment in the normal adnexal epithelium. These pigmented AKs were initially described as a clinical variant of AK with no other specific feature except the difficulty in distinguishing them from other pigmented lesions, on a morphological basis alone. However, the possibility that these lesions could represent a distinct clinicopathological entity with a marked progressive lateral spread compared with non-pigmented AK has been raised. Hence, the term 'spreading pigmented AK' (SPAK) was introduced. Typically, these SPAKs occur on the face. They are more than 1 cm in diameter and have a smooth, slightly scaly or verrucous surface.

Progressive lateral spread of these lesions may result in large areas of extensive actinic damage with various degree of brown-grey pigmentation. Definitive diagnosis of SPAK can be made only histologically.

The malignant potential of SPAK is not clearly known, but is likely to be the same as the classical AK. The progression of SPAK into squamous cell carcinoma has been described. An eventual transformation of SPAK into pigmented squamous cell carcinoma would seem logical, but the association of these two lesions has not yet been documented, probably because of lack of appropriate studies. No detailed electron microscopic study of the melanocytes and melanocyte–keratinocyte interactions in these lesions has been reported. Thus, the cause of the increased melanization in the SPAK is still unknown. The hypothesis that the dysplastic keratinocytes may in some way stimulate melanogenesis, melanosome production and melanosome transfer to them has been raised.

The differential diagnosis of pigmented spreading actinic keratosis must exclude actinic lentigo (senile lentigo), pigmented seborrhoeic keratosis, lentigo maligna (Dubreuilh's melanosis), lentigo maligna melanoma and melanocytic naevus. As the natural history and prognostic significance of these lesions differ considerably, awareness of the complete differential diagnosis with correct diagnosis of such pigmented lesions is of utmost importance. The clinical differentiation of these lesions is usually difficult and in many instances a definitive diagnosis can be made only histologically.

The treatment of pigmented AK or SPAK does not differ from that of classic non-pigmented AK, and includes cryosurgery, topical 5-fluorouracil and topical retinoids.

Pigmented basal cell epitheliomas

Increased pigmentation may occur in most morphological subtypes of basal cell carcinoma

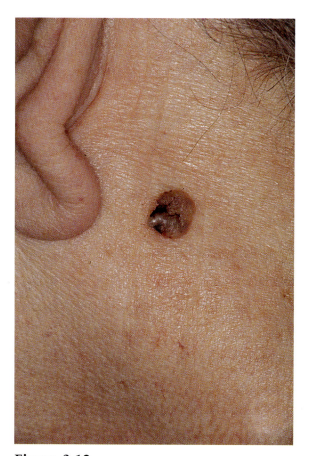

Figure 3.12

Hyperpigmented basal cell carcinoma.

with the possible exception of the morphoeic type. The most pigmented basal cell carcinomas are of the solid type (Figure 3.12). The uneven distribution of melanin within the tumour cells produces a blue-black colour, partly due to the deep situation of the pigment in the dermis. In most instances, the correct diagnosis is easy because the tumour, except for its pigmentation, bears all the typical clinical features of basal cell carcinoma.[11] However, in a few cases, the pigmented basal cell carcinoma may simulate a malignant melanoma.

Darkly pigmented basal cell carcinomas rarely develop in phototype I subjects. Histological examination demonstrates melanocytes interspersed among the tumour cells, which contain variable amounts of melanin granules. In addition, the lymphohistiocytic infiltrate contains large numbers of melanophages.

Pigmented squamous cell epitheliomas

Abundant melanin may be present within the cytoplasm of the neoplastic keratinocytes of pigmented squamous cell epitheliomas. This is produced by melanin-producing melanocytes that are scattered among the tumour cells, just as is the situation in pigmented basal cell carcinomas. These melanocytes transfer their pigment to surrounding neoplastic keratinocytes. Except for the hypermelanosis, these tumours have all the characteristic features of squamous cell carcinoma. Pigmented squamous cell epitheliomas are very uncommon.[11] Pigmented keratoacanthomas have been also described.

Erythrosis interfollicularis colli and poikiloderma of Civatte

Poikiloderma of Civatte is characterized by telangiectasia, atrophy and irregularity in pigmentation of the upper chest and lateral neck, but sparing the submental area.

In 1944, Leder[12] described an amazing skin disorder involving the lateral aspects of the neck, characterized clinically by a triad of erythema and telangiectasia, follicular papules and hyperpigmentation. It is likely that these two clinical phenotypes, respectively named erythrosis interfollicularis colli (EIC) and poikiloderma of Civatte, correspond to a single entity representing one of the skin manifestations of photoaging. It was initially thought that poikiloderma of Civatte was due to an imbalance in the endocrine system since it was most commonly observed in postmenopausal women. This clinical entity is now generally considered as an example of

Dyspigmentation and melanoma

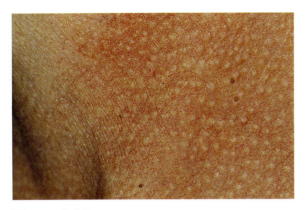

Figure 3.13
Poikiloderma of Civatte. Distinctive clinical picture with erythema, hyperpigmentation and follicular papules.

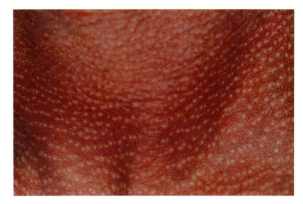

Figure 3.14
Poikiloderma of Civatte. Deep red erythema of the interfollicular areas.

photodamage that may occur in both men and women, although it is more common in middle-aged women. Very few reports on these skin disorders are available.[73]

The clinical picture is distinctive. Examination of the skin reveals a triad of symptoms comprising erythema and telangiectasia, follicular papules and hyperpigmentation. The red component between the follicular papules disappears with pressure, leaving only a brownish hue due to melanin pigmentation. The erythema may vary from pink to deep red. Close-up examination using a lens demonstrates a fine network of tiny telangiectatic blood vessels. Yellowish follicular micropapules are spread sometimes as longitudinal streaks on this erythematous background. The involved skin has been compared to a 'plucked chicken skin' (Figures 3.13 and 3.14). These pinhead-sized papules produce a granular texture on palpation. The topography of these lesions is also very distinctive. They are grouped in bilateral well-demarcated patches extending from the pre-auricular regions to the lateral aspects of the neck. The anterior borders of the affected areas are sharply delineated with sparing of the anterior submandibular zone appearing as a triangle of normal skin (Figure 3.15). Unilateral involvement has been reported in a few patients.

EIC may also involve the cheeks and the chin, and in rare cases the auricle, the eyebrows and the forehead. The lesions are usually asymptomatic. There is no evidence of scarring or atrophy. Moderate pruritus, a burning sensation in heat and an increase in perspiration in the affected area have also been described.

Histological features are not diagnostic but certain changes are commonly observed such as mild hyperkeratosis, follicular hyperplasia, follicular plugging, dilatation of superficial dermal blood vessels with minimal lymphocytic perivascular infiltration and melanin hyperpigmentation in the basal layer. Electron microscopic examination confirms the abundance of melanosomes both in melanocytes and keratinocytes, where most of them are found in the form of melanosome complexes.[14] Abnormally large melanosomes have been observed in one case.[14]

In reaching a diagnosis one needs to exclude Riehl's melanosis, érythrose péribuccale pigmentaire of Brocq, erythromelanosis

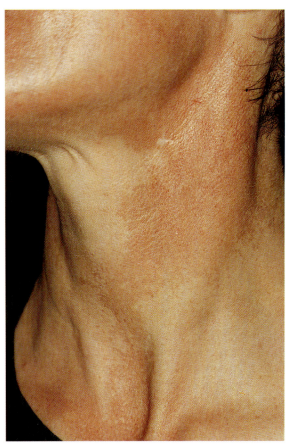

Figure 3.15

Poikiloderma of Civatte: typical distribution on the lateral aspects of the neck with sparing of the submental area.

suggests that chronic sun exposure plays a key role in this disorder. EIC usually begins in young adults and becomes more severe with age. Although the sun exposure time has not been evaluated in affected patients, the topography of the lesions in women, with involvement of the lateral aspects of the neck with sparing of the median submandibular area, strongly suggests a photoactive process. In some male patients, the sharp demarcation of the lesion at the border of the collar is an additional observation favouring this hypothesis. The involvement of additional factors such as phototoxic and/or photosensitizing agents in perfumes has also been discussed. Although EIC is mainly a cosmetic problem, this condition may be associated with serious psychological morbidity. Several topical treatments have been proposed, including tretinoin cream (0.05%), ammonium lactate cream and hydroquinone (2 or 3%), with some mild improvement. More recently, the use of pulsed yellow light from the flashlamp-pumped pulsed dye laser tuned at 585 nm has provided a successful form of therapy to remove both the telangiectasia and irregular pigmentation associated with poikiloderma of Civatte.[15] The pulsed-dye laser at 510 nm is also very useful in improving the pigmentary component of this disorder (personal observation).

Melanocyte naevogenesis

Photodamage may begin in young children. This is well illustrated by several epidemiological studies demonstrating that sun exposure plays a role in the development of melanocytic naevi in childhood.

Previous studies concluded that increased numbers of melanocytic naevi could be related to sunburn during childhood,[16] a tendency to burn rather than tan,[16] increased sun exposure,[16] proximity to the equator and holidays spent in a hot climate. On the other hand, some reports have not mentioned a

follicularis faciei, lichen pilaris faciei of Brocq, erythromelanosis follicularis faciei, lichen pilaris facici of Brocq, ulerythema ophryogenes and keratosis pilaris. However, the distribution and lack of clinical follicular keratosis readily distinguish erythromelanosis of the face and neck and poikiloderma of Civatte from the various forms of keratosis pilaris and from other facial melanoses.

Although most reports conclude that the aetiology and the pathogenesis of EIC and poikiloderma of Civatte are obscure, the original epidemiological study of Leder strongly correlation between sun exposure and melanocytic naevi. A recent study strongly supports a contribution of both acute and chronic sun exposure to the development of melanocytic naevi.[127] The finding of higher counts of melanocytic naevi on sun-exposed surfaces has provided further support for the role played by sun exposure in melanocytic naevogenesis. The number of melanocytic naevi in this population of 506 Australian children aged 1–6 years increased with age, probably as a consequence of cumulative lifetime sun exposure. The number of melanocytic naevi is considered as a risk factor for malignant melanoma.[5] If this is so, the pattern of melanoma risk seems to be established very early in life in children living in tropical regions.

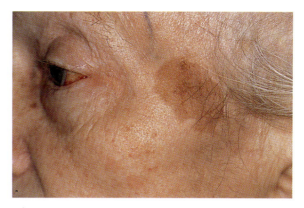

Figure 3.16

Dubreuilh's melanosis: clinically this lesion is sometimes difficult to differentiate from other pigmented lesions of facial skin in elderly individuals.

Dubreuilh's melanosis and lentigo maligna

Lentigo maligna (LM), also called Hutchinson's melanotic freckle or Dubreuilh's melanosis, is most commonly observed on the sun-exposed skin of the head and neck, particularly the face, with a predilection for the cheek, in an elderly patient. Arms, legs and trunk are rarely involved. Spreading of a cutaneous LM on to neighbouring mucosal surfaces such as the conjunctivae and oral mucosa may occur. LM develops generally in patients older than 40 years of age. The incidence increases progressively with age, with a mean age of 65 years, and peaks in the seventh and eighth decades of life. LM occurs almost exclusively in Caucasian subjects. There is a slight female preponderance in most large series. Clinically, the lesion presents as a slowly enlarging irregularly pigmented macule with areas of brown, black, pink or white colour and well-demarcated borders. Spontaneous regression rarely occurs. The size of the lesion varies from a few millimeters to several centimeters in diameter (Figure 3.16).

LM slowly increases in diameter. The radial growth phase of LM may last for 10–50 years before the development of a melanoma (LM melanoma, LMM). The lifetime risk of invasive melanoma in LM is unknown. Diagnosis of LM at 45 and 65 years of age gives the patient respectively a 47 per cent and 22 per cent lifetime risk of LMM.[18] Conversely, in one series of 85 pigmented lesions excised with a clinical diagnosis of LM more than 50 per cent had invasive LMM.

Malignant melanoma associated with LM is a darkly pigmented plaque or nodule superimposed on a circumscribed macule composed of various shades of higher and darker pigmentation, hypopigmentation and occasionally depigmentation (Figure 3.17).

Several studies suggest that, when controlled for depth of invasion and thickness, there is no difference in survival and local recurrence between LMM and the other malignant melanoma subtypes. Another report claimed that the 5-year survival rate for LMM was 90 per cent versus 66 per cent for the other groups of malignant melanoma, even though the LMMs were thicker.

Clinically, several facial pigmented lesions may be mistaken for LM. They include

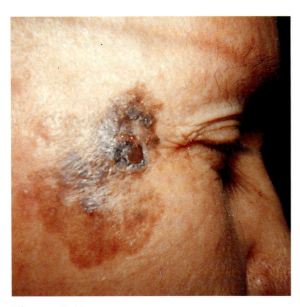

Figure 3.17

Malignant melanoma associated with Dubreuilh's melanosis.

from the changes induced by long-term UV exposure that include lentiginous melanocytic hyperplasia along the epidermal basement membrane. LM has a long, relatively benign clinical course. While some authors consider LM as an in situ malignant melanoma, others regard it as a premalignant melanocytic dysplasia.

Long-term cumulative UVR is believed to have a causative role. LM is postulated to develop from an abnormal clone of intraepidermal melanocytes on sun-damaged skin. Gene rearrangements of the 10q24–26 region of chromosome 10 [Et (10;11) (q26;p12)] and [t (9;10) (q22–q26)] have been detected in clones isolated from LM. X-radiation, oestrogen and progesterone, and non-permanent hair dyes appear to be associated with the development of LM, whereas cigarette smoking does not. LMM is most strongly linked to a relative or absolute inability to tan in response to UVR, to increased hours of sunlight, amount of actinic damage and a history of non-melanoma skin cancer.

Surgical excision with adequate margins of normal-appearing skin is probably the most reliable method of adequately removing LM. Conventional surgery for LM and LMM gives a 91 per cent cure rate (recurrences at a rate of 9 per cent developing within 14 months on average). Guidelines propose 1.0 cm margins for thin melanoma and this simple rule may be applied to LM. However, the histological margins of LM can extend further than the clinical lesions in many cases. In selected patients, Mohs' micrographic surgery aided by rush permanent sections may be used successfully. This technique offers the ability to detect subclinical disease in those lesions that extend beyond the clinical margin, and gives a higher cure rate than conventional surgery. In elderly patients other therapeutic options, such as cryotherapy, Grenz-irradiation, topical 5-fluorouracil, dermabrasion, ionizing radiation and laser therapy with CO_2, argon or the various 'pigmented' lasers, have been employed. However, these destructive treatment modali-

pigmented solar lentigo, junctional naevus, seborrhoeic keratosis, pigmented actinic keratoses and pigmented epitheliomas.

Histologically, LM is characterized by an increased number of cytologically atypical melanocytes in the basal layers of an atrophic epidermis overlying solar elastotic sun-damaged dermis. Atypical melanocytes, sometimes multinucleated, arranged along the epidermal basal layer in solitary units or small nests, can extend far beyond the clinical margin of the lesion. Periadnexal extension of atypical melanocytes in the follicular outer root sheath and eccrine duct is also a common feature of LM. In addition, a dense infiltration of the upper dermis by melanin-laden melanophages is usually observed. The histological diagnosis for LM must exclude conditions such as benign melanocytic neoplasms, for example naevocellular naevius, pigmented actinic keratosis or pigmented seborrhoeic keratosis. LM may be difficult to distinguish

Dyspigmentation and melanoma

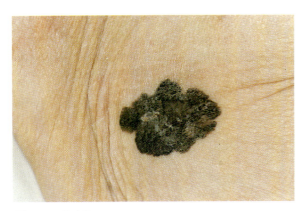

Figure 3.18
Superficial spreading melanoma.

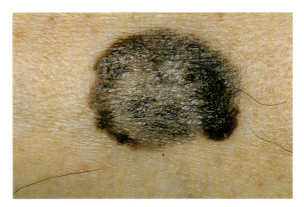

Figure 3.19
Superficial spreading melanoma demonstrating a typical colour variegation.

ties are associated with high recurrence rates. Cryotherapy is theoretically effective due to increased sensitivity of melanocytes to cryodestruction, although recurrence rates as high as 50 per cent have been reported. Radiation therapy, including Grenz-irradiation, topical application of radium, insertion of radon seeds and electron beam radiation, have also been used. Poor results and high recurrence rates have been observed with curettage, dermabrasion and electrodessication. The various laser treatments have had minimal success in treating LM.[19] Good to excellent results have been reported in a few cases treated with 15 or 20 per cent azelaic acid cream, but this approach has a significant failure rate and cannot be recommended as standard treatment for LM. Topical 5-fluorouracil treatment alone gives very limited success but is useful in combination with surgical excision. Topical hydroquinone and topical tretinoin are not effective in the treatment of LM.

Melanomas

From the clinical point of view, four variants of cutaneous melanoma may be distinguished. The flat melanoma corresponding to histologically superficial spreading melanoma is the commonest of the melanomas. It may be found anywhere on the skin. It is a pigmented lesion, with its greatest diameter usually exceeding 5 mm (Figures 3.18 and 3.19).

Nodular melanoma may appear on healthy skin on any part of the body. It presents as an elevated or polypoid lesion. It may be uniform in pigmentation and frequently shows ulceration when advanced. LMM occurs as a macular lesion on sun-exposed skin (head, neck) and is common in elderly patients. Acral lentiginous melanoma presents as a darkly pigmented flat to nodular lesion on palms and soles or subungually.

Several clinical features of malignant melanoma are helpful for differentiating benign and malignant pigmented lesions and thus allowing early detection, the key to favourable prognosis. They include assymetry, border irregularity, colour variegation, and diameter ≥6 mm.[20] An 'assymetric' lesion is one that is not regularly round or oval. A line cannot be drawn through the centre of the lesion to bisect it into halves that appear almost exactly the same. The 'border irregularity' refers to notching, scalloping and

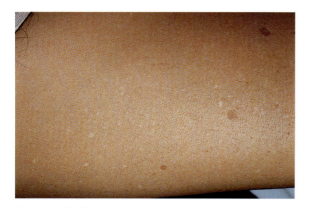

Figure 3.20

Idiopathic guttate hypomelanosis. Typical distribution of small hypomelanotic macules on the limbs.

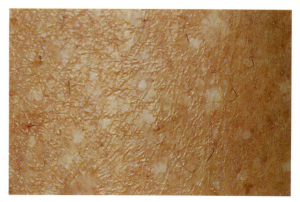

Figure 3.21

Close view of idiopathic guttate hypomelanosis lesions demonstrating the absence of scarring and atrophy.

poorly defined lesion margins. 'Colour variegation' refers to a pigmented lesion with various areas of brown, tan, red, white or blue-black, or a combination thereof. Although a high suspicion exists for a lesion ≥6 mm in diameter, early melanoma may be diagnosed at a smaller size.

There is abundant evidence suggesting a causal relationship between UV radiation and development of melanoma. The great majority of melanomas in light-skinned people are due to UV radiation and at least at moderate total levels of exposure, intermittent relatively intense exposure of unacclimatized skin is the major risk factor for the more common types of melanoma, superficial spreading melanomas and nodular melanoma.[21] Estimates suggest that at least 65 per cent of cutaneous melanomas worldwide are caused by sun exposure.[22] Recent studies suggest that the number of melanocytic naevi that develop by the age of 20 is influenced by cumulative sun exposure from birth as well as severe childhood sunburns and fair skin phenotype. Furthermore, an increased number of melanocytic naevi is an important risk factor for the development of melanoma.[23] Melanoma should be preventable by a reduction in sun exposure and by a specific effort to avoid intermittent intense exposure, particularly in early childhood.

Save for LMM, malignant melanoma rarely occurs on the most sun-exposed parts of the body such as the face, where photoaging is most prominent. Thus a direct and simple relationship between photoaging and malignant melanoma other than LMM is unlikely. The role of solar exposure in the induction of cutaneous malignant melanoma cannot be simply interpreted on the cumulative role of UV irradiation and implicates more complex aetiological mechanisms.[24]

Hypomelanotic lesions

Idiopathic guttate hypomelanosis

This disorder characterized by multiple small discrete pure white macules is almost specifically distributed on the sun-exposed surfaces of the forearms and legs, usually in association with other skin changes of chronological

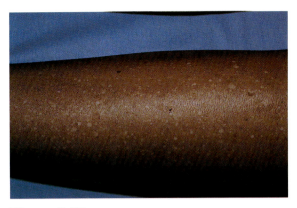

Figure 3.22

Characteristic small size of idiopathic guttate hypomelanosis lesions.

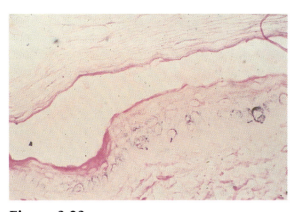

Figure 3.23

Idiopathic guttate hypomelanosis (light microscopy). Irregular melanin pigmentation in the epidermal basal layer.

aging and photodamage. Idiopathic guttate hypomelanosis (IGH) provokes cosmetic discomfort. Furthermore, most physicians do not recognize this asymptomatic disorder and confuse it with vitiligo or some form of cutaneous depigmentation induced by pityriasis.

IGH is a very common disorder. Its incidence ranges from 47 per cent up to 68 per cent among patients and visitors of dermatology clinics. Although originally reported in black individuals, this dermatosis is seen in all races. In Caucasoids, it occurs among patients of all hair and eye colours, but there seems to be a preponderance among those with brown eyes and brown hair. Males and females are probably equally affected. Several studies suggest a female predominance, but this apparent increase is probably the result of a heightened perception of a cosmetic problem by women compared with men. IGH is a disease of adults and senescence; although onset has been reported in children as young as 5 years, epidemiological studies strongly support an increased incidence of the condition with age. Furthermore, the number of lesions increases with age, and also after excessive sun exposure.

The typical IGH lesion is a circumscribed, sharply defined, porcelain white macule (Figure 3.20).[25] The lesions may be delineated by the skin furrows. They are also characterized by small size (usually from 0.2 mm to 6 mm with occasional larger lesions up to 1.5 cm). Once present these lesions do not change in size, and are not confluent. Their surface is smooth, not infiltrated, without scarring and atrophy (Figure 3.21). No spontaneous repigmentation has been observed. Vellus hair within the lesions usually retains their pigment. The lesions are quite easily visible with standard illumination, but Wood's light increases the contrast between involved and surrounding normal skin. In most patients, multiple white macules are present (several to ten, sometimes more than 50) (Figure 3.22).

The white macules are usually distributed in the sun-exposed surface of the extremities, with no involvement of the sun-protected skin in most patients. Involvement of abdominal and facial skin has been reported. The depigmented macules are asymptomatic.

The most consistent histopathological features of the white macules are a flattening of the dermal–epidermal junction, moderate

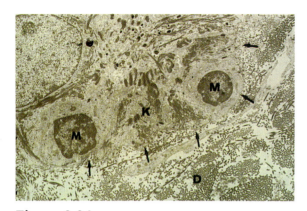

Figure 3.24

Idiopathic guttate hypomelanosis (electron microscopy). Melanocytes with little or no melanogenic activity may be present in the lesions.

to marked reduction or focal absence of the melanin granules in the basal and suprabasal layers, and a basketweave hyperkeratosis (Figure 3.23). Less frequent features include increased collagen or elastic fibres, slight pigmentary incontinence, slightly thickened and fibrotic papillary dermis, elastorrhexis, collagen homogenization and collagen basophilia. Interestingly, some of these histological features are also found in photodamaged skin. There is a moderate to relatively marked reduction in the number of dopa-positive epidermal melanocytes (10–50 per cent when compared with normal skin), but these cells are never totally absent, even in hypomelanotic skin. At the ultrastructural level, some of these melanocytes have normal melanogenic activity. Some others have abundant cytoplasm but lack mature melanosomes, having a predominance of stage I and II immature forms (Figure 3.24). The keratinocytes show a marked variation in melanin content, which may be absent or markedly decreased. The epidermal basement membrane and the dermal component show no special alterations. Thus, in contrast to vitiligo, the epidermal melanocytes are present in IGH lesions.

The diagnosis of IGH can usually be readily established on a clinical basis and skin biopsy for histological examination is not required. Conditions which must be excluded on diagnosis include such hypopigmentary disorders as vitiligo, lichen sclerosus atrophie blanche en plaque, hypomelanotic guttate parapsoriasis, achromic pityriasis versicolor, achromic planar warts, pityriasis alba, leprosy, syphilis, and chemical and postinflammatory hypopigmentation. Confetti-like hypomelanosis of the legs, very similar to IGH, has also been observed in a mother and son with tuberous sclerosis.[26]

Recently, disseminated hypopigmented keratoses have been reported as a newly recognized dermatologic entity.[27] This disorder is closely related and most likely identical to IGH.

The cause of IGH is unknown, but several arguments suggest that it results at least partly from chronic natural UV light exposure.

- IGH lesions occur on the more exposed areas of the upper and lower extremities following the pattern of most photosensitive dermatoses (extensor aspect of the limbs). In contrast, the protected zones are relatively free of hypomelanotic macules.
- IGH is more frequently observed in female patients with a history of chronic sun exposure.
- IGH-like lesions have been described in PUVA-treated patients with psoriasis or mycosis fungoides. An epidemiological study concluded that no significant difference in terms of actinic exposure time expressed in hours during a lifetime period was observed between the IGH patients and the normal controls.[28] No differences were observed in clinical scores of skin photodamage between the affected subjects and the normal individuals, suggesting a lack of relationship between coexisting actinic damage and the presence of IGH lesions. None of

these arguments is strong enough to rule out a causative role for sun exposure.

An interesting experiment suggests that there is an active depigmenting mechanism in IGH. In two subjects with IGH, exchange grafts from normal to hypomelanotic skin and vice versa were performed and observed during 1.5 years.[28] The normally pigmented grafts progressively lost their pigmentation, whereas the achromic implants not only kept their leukodermic condition but grew slightly.

Chronological aging with gradual loss of active melanocytes has been proposed as a cause of IGH. This hypothesis does not explain the characteristic sun-exposed distribution of IGH. Autoimmunity has also been suggested as a pathogenic factor for IGH but there are very few data to support this view. The lack of scarring in IGH lesions makes the hypothesis of a traumatic factor leading to a residual hypopigmentation very unlikely.

No effective treatment is yet available. Oral PUVA therapy (20 mg 8-MOP (8-methoxypsozalen) daily for 2 months, plus sunlight) has been tried in one patient. An estimated two-thirds repigmentation was observed. Cessation of treatment was followed by a gradual loss of pigment. Photochemistry or phototherapy should not be proposed for the treatment of IGH as it is itself most likely a clinical manifestation of photodamage.

Intralesional triamcinolone alone (2 mg/ml injected every month for 3 months) has been used with a good and statistically significant response in about half of the patients. However, this treatment cannot be advocated as a therapeutic approach for IGH,[28] due to the risk of atrophy and hypomelanosis which it involves. Another study[29] suggests that cryotherapy with liquid nitrogen could be a treatment of IGH. Lesions gently frozen (application of a cryoprobe for 10 seconds) repigmented in 6–8 weeks. During the first week after treatment, all cryotreated lesions blistered. During the third week, perifollicular repigmentation was observed. Complete repigmentation was obtained in 90.8 per cent of the lesions. Histological study of the repigmenting lesions demonstrated the reappearance of dopa-positive melanocytes. The authors suggest that liquid nitrogen destroys all melanocytes and keratinocytes in IGH lesions and induces an epidermal wound healing with migration of surrounding normal melanocytes into IGH skin. Although no side-effects are mentioned, the risk of hypo- or secondary-hypermelanosis should be considered.

In general, the cosmetic disfigurement is usually mild. As sunlight is most likely a precipitating factor, sunbathing should be discouraged and use of topical sunscreens with high sun protection factors strongly recommended.

Stellate spontaneous pseudoscars

Clinically, spontaneous stellate pseudoscars (SSPs) appear as small white spots, non- or only slightly protruding, and usually located on the back of the hands or on the extensor aspects of forearms (Figure 3.25).[30] They are rarely seen elsewhere. Although their forms vary, they have a stellate shape in their most characteristic form. These lesions are very common and mainly appear after 60 years of age, and become particularly frequent after 70 years. In 500 people studied at between 70 and 90 years of age, SSPs were found to be multiplying slowly with time.

These lesions develop in patients with a diffuse senile skin atrophy. They are often associated with Bateman's purpura. Histological studies show that SSPs are composed of a small mass of fibrous connective tissue directly beneath the epidermis in which elastic fibers are lacking or severely damaged. The whitish appearance of these lesions may suggest a defect in the melanocyte system of the skin. No specific histochemical or ultrastructural study of the melanocytes in SSPS has yet been performed, but specific stains for melanins show that the epidermis is

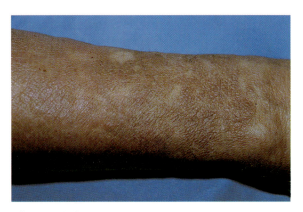

Figure 3.25
Stellate spontaneous pseudoscars are usually located on the extensor aspects of forearms.

normally pigmented. This suggests that the white colour is not due to a melanocyte defect, but rather to dermal abnormalities.

The pathogenesis of SSP is not clear. The role of repeated microtrauma has been suggested but never demonstrated. The patients' histories strongly suggest that this pseudoscar appears spontaneously, although some indicate that injury occurred. The localization of SSPs suggests a predisposing role of chronic sun exposure. The occurrence of presenile forms of SSP in younger patients with extensive sun exposure and pellagroid changes related to alcoholism and in patients with albinism further support this hypothesis. Other causes of presenile SSP include corticosteroid treatments.

Although protein anabolic agents and vitamin E have been tried, no effective treatment is presently available.

Dyspigmentation of chronological aging

Decrease in the number of epidermal dopa-positive melanocytes

The number of dopa-positive melanocytes in human skin decreases with age by approximately 10–20 per cent with each decade.[31] This is observed in both habitually sun-exposed and protected areas. Melanocyte density, however, is approximately twofold higher in chronically sun-exposed skin than in protected skin at all ages.[32] From these results, Gilchrest et al[32] suggested that the principal effect of chronic sun exposure on human epidermal melanocytes is not premature aging but activation and/or proliferation of the exposed melanocytes. Repeated UV irradiation of non-exposed melanocytes on the buttocks, for example, increases the number of melanocytes even in old subjects.[31] The higher numbers of epidermal melanocytes in sun-exposed human skin may be explained by repeated exposure irreversibly increasing the number of dopa-positive melanocytes. All these quantitative studies on melanocyte populations have been performed using the dopa reaction, a technique that identifies melanocytes by their melanogenic activity, but cannot differentiate between a change in number of melanocytes and a loss in dopa-oxidase activity. It would be useful, therefore, to compare exposed and protected skin using probes that are not related to the melanogenic activity of the pigment cells.

Very few in vitro studies have been performed to explain age-associated changes in melanocytes. Preliminary studies suggest that melanocytes derived from adult skin have a considerably shorter life span in vitro, with decreased response to specific mitogens.[32]

Changes in the number of melanocytic naevi

'If we could all live to be over ninety, we could probably depart from life as we enter it, free of moles.'' This statement by Stegmaier[33] is confirmed by many epidemiological studies which demonstrate age-related changes in melanocytic naevi (MN). MNs are very seldom present at birth. In a large series of newborn infants they were found in only 1 per cent of those examined. These lesions develop later in childhood, adolescence and early adulthood. MNs are almost universally present in young adults. The peak incidence of MNs is usually observed during the second and third decades. The average number per person in this age group ranges from 15 to 40. There is a significant association between skin complexion phenotype and number of moles. Subjects with light complexion have higher mean counts of MNs than those with a dark complexion. Later, there is a progressive decrease in the number of these lesions.

The median number of MNs in people over 50 has been estimated to be 3.2 per person with no important changes between 50 and 80. Other studies demonstrate that MNs are rarely present in persons over the age of 80 years. This suggests that MNs involute. Thus, the life cycle of MNs is as follows: a growth phase from birth until young adulthood followed by a relatively long period of quiescence and eventual involution after 50 years of age.

The mechanism by which MNs disappear is not known. Histological studies demonstrate that both junctional proliferation and total cellularity of naevi decrease with age. In addition, naevus cells within the dermis are replaced by connective tissue elements, demonstrating that aging of MNs is associated with changes between the melanocytic component and the stroma.

Hyperpigmented seborrhoeic keratoses

Seborrhoeic keratosis (SK) is a common benign tumour of the skin with accentuated melanin pigmentation, also known as a senile wart, seborrheic wart and basal cell papilloma. SK usually develops in people over forty. According to a recent study,[34] the frequency of SK is increasing. The studies also show an increasing frequency of SK with age. The prevalence of SK ranges from 12% in

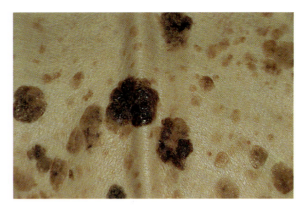

Figure 3.26

Typical hyperpigmented seborrhoeic keratoses.

15–25 year olds to 100% of those aged over 50 years. Furthermore, in patients with lesions, the median number of lesions also increases with age from six per person in 15–25 years.[34] The prevalence and numbers of lesions per person does not differ between men and women. SK have been reported to be less common in populations with dark skin compared with those with white skin. Epidemiological data suggest that exposure to sunlight is a risk factor for SK. Indeed, SKs on exposed areas are more often flat and more than 3 mm greater in diameter than those in the non-exposed areas. Although absolute numbers of SK are higher on the trunk, when taking into account body surface areas, they are more concentrated on the areas frequently exposed to sunlight i.e. the head and neck and dorsum of each hand.[34]

SKs typically begin as flat macules with sharply demarcated borders. Their surface has a characteristic rough or verrucous appearance with multiple plugged follicles (Figure 3.26). SK may vary in colour from yellow to pale-brown with pink tones or to dark-brown or black (Figure 3.27). These lesions can appear on any part of the body except the mucous membranes but they occur more commonly on the face and trunk. SK result

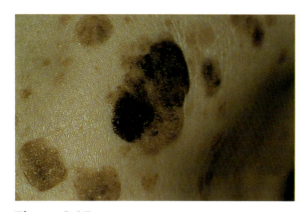

Figure 3.27
The degree of hyperpigmentation varies considerably from one seborrhoeic keratosis to another.

from epidermal proliferation and from thickening of the papillary dermis. Many SKs have an increased amount of melanin within their keratinocytes varying from moderate to abundant. Melanin is present mostly in the basaloid cells, but may also be found in macrophages in the upper part of the dermis. Immunohistochemistry reveals the occurrence of many DOPA-positive melanocytes in the basal layer of the lesions.[35]

The pathogenesis of SKs is unknown. There may be a genetic predisposition for these lesions. Sun exposure may play a role in their development and increased constitutive melanin pigmentation of the skin may be a protective factor against their occurrence. Although the molecular mechanisms underlying the keratinocyte hyperproliferation and the increased melanin production occurring in these lesions are not understood, a recent study suggests that endothelin-1 plays a key-role in these processes.[35] Endothelin-1 is a strong mitogen and melanogen for human melanocytes. UVB exposure stimulates autocrine production of ET-1 in keratinocytes leading to the paracrine activation of melanocyte function as seen in UVB hyperpigmentation. In SKs highly melanogenic melanocytes are localized generally in the vicinity of proliferating ET-1 positive keratinocytes. Furthermore, RT-PCR of the RNA isolated from the lesional skin of SK reveals a markedly increased expression of the tyrosinase and the ET-1 genes. These mRNA signals are undetectable in perilesional skin of SKs. Thus, it is likely that the accentuated secretion of ET-1 in SKs is responsible for the increased melanin pigmentation of SKs.

SKs respond well to liquid nitrogen cryotherapy. Other treatment modalities include curettage and light electrodessication.

Greying and whitening of hair

Greying of hair is the physical trait most closely correlating with chronological age of all physiological functions (Figure 3.28). This very common phenomenon occurs to a varying degree in all persons. No race or sex is spared, but the age of onset varies among several populations. The age of onset seems largely inherited, but other factors are probably involved. Usually, greying of hair begins in the late fourth or early fifth decade, but onset in the twenties or early thirties is not uncommon.[25]

Grey hair usually appears first at the temples and slowly extends to the vertex and later to the remainder of the scalp. Beard and body are usually involved later. Chest, pubic and axillary hairs may retain their pigment even in old age. Greying of hair is usually irreversible but a few cases of reversal of greying have been reported.

Although there are still some controversies, most investigators agree that the number of melanocytes in grey hair is greatly reduced. A marked vacuolization of pigment cells has also been described. The number of melanosomes in keratinocytes is decreased and most of the pigment granules show abnormal structural features. Clearly senile greying is related to a decreased number of active melanocytes and decreased melanogenic activity of the remain-

Dyspigmentation and melanoma

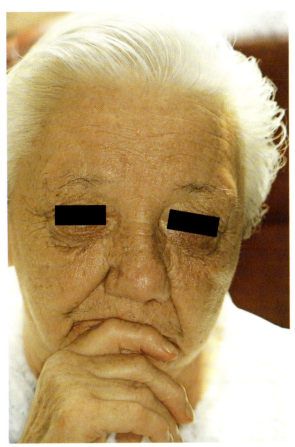

Figure 3.28
Typical whitening of hair with chronological aging.

ing melanocytes. The mechanism underlying this decrease is not firmly established. Is it destruction or loss of dopa-oxidase activity?)

The precise cause of senile greying of hair has not been established. Although normally present in pigmented human scalp hair follicles, α-melanocyte-stimulating hormone binding sites are absent in senile white hair follicles.[36] The role of some disturbance of immune tolerance has been suggested, but little evidence supports this idea. Animal models of senile greying of hair include guinea pigs, rats, rabbits, dogs, sheep and horses. A progressive loss of hair pigmentation inherited as an autosomal dominant trait and influenced by unspecified maternal effects has been described in wild-type Australian mice. This suggested that heredity is a significant factor. Hair melanocytes may have their own genetically determined internal clock for development and resolution. Greying with age has also been described in mice infected endogenously or exogenously with murine leukaemia virus. From an ultrastructural study demonstrating that amelanotic hairs contain clear cells resembling the melanocytes present in hair bulbs of albino mice, it was suggested that the process of greying with age was the result of melanocyte dysfunction rather than loss. The possibility that melanocytes are susceptible to virus infection at a critical stage of differentiation and that virus expression could interfere with cellular functions at some later stage of melanocyte development was also raised.

Several experimental findings suggest that some of the intermediate metabolites of the melanin pathway have a cytotoxic activity. It may be hypothesized that a progressive loss of some natural protective mechanisms of senile hair follicle melanocytes results in destruction of pigment cells. Recent studies suggest that such mechanisms could be responsible for premature greying in light (B^{lt}) mice. In these animals, the hair is pigmented at the tip but very lightly or not at all pigmented at the base due to clumping, irregular distribution, and reduced number of melanosomes followed by premature death of follicular melanocytes. This phenotype occurs only in pigmented mice, suggesting that it may be mediated through the inherent cytotoxicity of pigment production.[37] It is the result of a single base alteration at the brown mouse locus coding for the TRP-1. The function of TRP-1 is not yet known, but this observation suggests that it plays a critical role in the stabilization of melanosome structure.

Transgenic Bcl-2-deficient mice may represent an interesting model of greying of hair.

The initial hair pigmentation of these animals on a black coat colour background is indistinguishable from that of their normal littermates during the first hair follicle cycle. When these initial hairs are replaced during the second follicle cycle, the coat of Bcl-2-deficient mice becomes markedly hypopigmented.[38] Melanin staining documented the presence of melanin in all hairs of these mice, suggesting that a decrease in dark pigment rather than a loss of melanocytes accounts for this greying. The Bcl-2 gene inhibits most types of apoptotic cell death by regulating an antioxidant pathway at sites of free radical generation. Thus, it is likely that the greying of hair is due to a defect in redox-regulated melanin synthesis. Whether the light mouse and the Bcl-2-deficient mice are valuable models for the study of senile and premature greying of hair in man remains to be established.

Pathogenesis

The modifications of the epidermal melanocyte population induced by chronic exposure to UV radiation involve changes in both cell proliferation and differentiation. The higher melanocyte density in chronically sun-exposed skin compared with protected skin suggests that repeated UV exposure induces a dysregulation of epidermal melanocyte homeostasis. The molecular events underlying these effects have not been clearly identified and very little is known regarding the mechanisms by which UV light affects the cell cycle machinery of human melanocytes. UV irradiation causes a chain of molecular and cellular changes in the skin that affect all cells, in particular melanocytes.

Although one report concludes that ultraviolet B radiation (UVB) acts as an independent mitogen for normal human melanocytes in culture, several studies have demonstrated that cultured melanocytes respond with growth inhibition to multiple irradiations with UV light. After UVB irradiations, melanocytes are blocked in G1.[39] This ability of UVB-irradiated melanocytes to enter into S-phase correlates with prolonged overexpression of the p53 protein and the cyclin-dependent kinase inhibitor p21 Waf-1/Cip-1/SDJ-1. Further UVB irradiation inhibits the phosphorylation of the retinoblastoma tumour suppressor gene product Rb, and delays the expression of the proliferating cell nuclear antigen (PCNA), but does not induce activation of the microtubule associated protein (MAP)-kinase pathway.

After UV-irradiation, keratinocytes are known to synthesize a variety of cytokines, including IL-1, IL-6, IL-8, tumour necrosis factor-α and transforming growth factor-β, that may have a direct effect on melanocyte proliferation and survival. The production of basic fibroblast growth factor, the best-characterized keratinocyte-produced melanocyte mitogen,[40] is increased by UVB exposure.

Cultured human keratinocytes synthesize and secrete endothelin-1. The production of this factor is also increased after UVB irradiation in a dose-dependent manner. Endothelin derivatives stimulate the proliferation and melanization of human melanocytes via a receptor-mediated signal transduction pathway.[41] Similar findings have been observed for nerve growth factor. These studies suggest that these keratinocyte-derived factors may play an essential role in the maintenance of melanocyte proliferation and perhaps in the pathogenesis of dyspigmentation of photoaged skin.[42]

In addition to photoaging of melanocytes, chronic UV exposure of melanocytes plays an important role in melanocyte carcinogenesis. Chronic growth stimulation of melanocytes by leukotriene C4 induces pleiotropic modifications in the normal melanocyte phenotype. These findings not only suggest that inflammatory mediators have a role in human epidermal melanocytes but provide insight into alteration of melanocyte growth which may have relevance in melanocyte photoaging and in early stages of melanocyte oncogenesis.[43] It is likely that the well-known effects of UVR on skin cells, such as direct DNA damage and thymine dimerization, and production of oxidative free radicals (e.g. superoxide anion and hydroxyl radicals), also play a critical role in the pathogenesis of melanocyte photoaging.[44]

The phenotype of epidermal melanocytes of photoaged skin, such as those present in actinic lentigo, has not yet been characterized. Such studies should be most informative in helping us to understand the progression of melanocyte photoaging.

Treatment

Topical tretinoin

Several clinical studies demonstrate that topical tretinoin improves the irregular hyperpigmentation associated with photoaging.[45] This effect is dose-dependent.[46] A significant lightening of hyperpigmented lesions associated with photodamage in patients treated for 10 months with once daily application of 0.1% all-*trans*-retinoic acid (RA) cream has been reported.[47] Of a group of 24 patients with actinic lentigines of the face who were treated with tretinoin, 20 experienced lightening of these lesions as compared with 8 of 28 patients with facial lesions who received vehicle. The results for lesions of the upper extremities were similar. There were no recurrences during a 6-month follow-up period after discontinuation of therapy. These included actinic lentigines and non-lentiginous lesions. A statistically significant reduction in epidermal melanin pigmentation was observed in these two types of lesion.[47] However, there was no change in the number and size of melanocytes. Furthermore, the degree of clubbing of rete ridges, a modification associated with actinic lentigines, was not changed at the end of treatment. Asian individuals with photoaging primarily have hyperpigmented lesions and only a small degree of wrinkling after years of sun exposure[48] These lesions correspond to actinic lentigines and to non-lentiginous lesions including pigmented seborrhoeic keratoses, benign keratoses, solar elastosis and spongiotic dermatitis. All investigations on Asiatics have consistently shown that topical 0.05% or 0.1% RA cream for 6–12 months improves hyperpigmented spots.[49]

This lightening is obtained for hyperpigmented spots on both the face and the hands.[49] After several months of treatment, there is a statistically significant decrease in epidermal pigmentation in the tretinoin group compared with the control group.[49] The lentiginous downgrowths with increased hypertrophic melanocytes, observed before treatment, had practically disappeared after 12 months of daily use of topical tretinoin.[50]

The mechanism of action of tretinoin on these pigmentary abnormalities of photoaged skin has not yet been elucidated. After RA treatment, the size and number of epidermal melanocytes decreased.[45] In a 24-week study using three different tretinoin concentrations, a significant dose-dependent decrease in the epidermal melanin content was observed. This modification was apparently stable, the decreased epidermal melanin content being still present after 48 weeks of tretinoin treatment, while other histological changes such as stratum corneum compaction, increased epidermal thickness and increased granular layer thickness returned to baseline. Only a 0.001% tretinoin treatment showed no effect on melanin pigmentation. This observation may suggest that there was a decrease in the melanogenic activity of melanocytes after RA treatment. The ultrastructural demonstration that in photoaged skin after topical tretinoin melanocytes had fewer dendritic processes and fewer and more immature melanosomes also supports this view. Various hypotheses have been proposed, such as a decrease of melanosome transfer to keratinocytes, secondary to an increased epidermal turnover. This is further suggested by the effect of topical tretinoin on a pigment macule reassembling human freckles that occurs on the face of macaques.[51] The hyperpigmentation is due to an epidermal hypermelanosis with an increased number of 'well-developed' dopa-positive melanocytes. Interestingly, topical 0.1% tretinoin has been shown to induce a significant depigmentation of this lesion, as early as 1 month after commencing treatment. Morphological studies have not been able to demonstrate any changes in the size, number and melanogenic activity of melanocytes, despite a marked reduction of epidermal melanin pigmentation. As the number of S-phase basal cells has been shown to increase by approximately 50 per cent after tretinoin treatment, it has been suggested that RA-induced lightening of the macules may be largely due to the dispersion of melanin granules in acanthotic keratinocytes and their fast turnover.[51] However, this is probably too simplistic a view and it is not yet established whether these effects of RA on photoaged skin result from its direct effect on melanocytes or from an indirect action via keratinocytes and/or keratinocyte-derived factors, or via dermal influences. Another noteworthy observation is that topical 0.1% tretinoin appears to stimulate melanogenesis in the Yucatan pig.[52] Electron microscopy has revealed an increase in the number and size of melanocytes in tretinoin-treated areas of skin. The melanosomes are also larger and more abundant within the melanocytes and keratinocytes. The reason for this disparity between the response of the human and the pig skin is not yet known. Clinical trials have shown that topical tretinoin can modify dysplastic or malignant melanocytes. Fading of some lesions or elimination of some dysplastic naevi with histological evidence of disappearance or reversion to benign naevi has been reported following tretinoin treatment.[53] The daily application of a 0.05% tretinoin solution for 4 months to cutaneous melanoma metastases induced significant regression in two patients. These observations, which are of no practical value for the treatment of these pigmented lesions, suggest a definite biological effect of topical tretinoin on pigment cells.[53]

Only a few studies carried out to elucidate the action of RA on the proliferation and melanogenic activity of pigment cells have been reported. They have been performed on melanoma cells, and it is difficult to extrapolate the results to normal human melanocytes. Despite these limitations, these studies can help us understand the effects of RA on the melanin pigmentary system in humans.[54]

Retinoic acid and melanogenesis in pigment cells

In vitro studies

Several biochemical studies have been performed on different melanoma cell lines and normal human melanocytes in vitro to evaluate the effect of retinoids or RA on melanin synthesis. RA has been reported as either a stimulator or suppressor of basal melanization in these cells.[55,56]

The main conclusion to be drawn from the study of melanoma cells is that RA affects melanogenesis via a direct effect on pigment cells. However, due to the specific reactivity of each cell line, it is difficult to conclude that there is an unequivocal effect of RA on the melanogenic activity of these cells.

Few data are at present available on the effects of RA on normal human melanocytes. In a recent review by Yaar and Gilchrest,[57] it is stated that retinoids have not been demonstrated to have any effect in these cells. When treated with RA, epidermal melanocytes grown in a serum-free culture medium which was supplemented with fibroblast growth factor, bovine pituitary extract, insulin and phorbol myristate acetate did not display significant changes in either the melanin content or tyrosinase activity. More recent data establish that melanocyte density affects the RA response in cultured human melanocytes. At subconfluent density of melanocytes, RA increases tyrosinase activity and melanogenesis, whereas at confluent density RA inhibits tyrosine activity and new melanin formation. As the total activity of protein kinase C (PKC) is higher at confluent than at subconfluent density, it may be suggested that melanocyte density may affect melanogenesis, perhaps by modulating the level of the PKC isoform required to activate tyrosinase, as well as the ability of the enzyme to respond to RA. Another study demonstrates that *cis*- and *trans*-RA significantly decrease the UVB-stimulated melanogenesis (tyrosinase activity and melanin neosynthesis) in mouse melanoma cells and in normal human melanocytes.[58] RA inhibition of UVB-induced melanogenesis acts at the post-transcriptional level, leading to a decreased tyrosinase and tyrosinase related protein (TRP-1) synthesis. On the other hand, inhibition of TRP-2 following UVB treatment of normal human melanocytes is significantly reversed by RA.

In vivo studies

Topically applied all-*trans*-retinoic acid (0.5 mg/ml in a solvent consisting of ethanol dimethylsulphoxide and acetone) greatly enhances UV radiation-induced melanogenesis in lightly pigmented mice (skh: HR-2), which are able to develop a tan. This observation was confirmed in two human volunteers.[59] In keeping with these observations, recent data suggest that topical retinoic acid (0.1% for 4 days under occlusion) induces tyrosinase activity in normal non-sun-exposed skin of white subjects in vivo.[60] In black skin, in vivo, high tyrosinase activity was not associated with increased tyrosinase mRNA or protein levels, indicating that regulation of tyrosinase activity by RA occurs at a post-translational level. These observations raise the possibility that long-term RA treatment may produce increased melanin content in human skin.

Retinoic acids, retinoids and proliferation of pigment cells

RA inhibits proliferation of B16 mouse melanoma cells, murine S91 C^2 cells and K-1735P cells.[61]

In the human melanoma cell lines SK Mel-28 and A 375, exposure to RA resulted in a complete lack of any antiproliferative activity, but acritretin exposure produced only a low-grade inhibition of growth in one of these two cell lines. By contrast, other retinoids (isotretinoin, temaroten, Ro 13-7410, Ro 13-6307 and Ro 14-6113) inhibited growth by 50 per cent in this system. Proliferation of normal human melanocytes grown in serum-free culture medium was also inhibited by RA.

The mechanism by which RA induces growth inhibition in B16 melanoma cells in vitro has been further examined. RA induced PKC in these cells. RA also increased the amount of cyclic AMP-dependent protein kinase. The recent finding that B16 mouse melanoma cells selected for resistance for growth inhibition mediated by cyclic AMP were cross-resistant to retinoic acid-induced growth inhibition suggested that cyclic AMP regulates some step in the RA signal transduction pathway in these cells.[62]

Retinoic acid and migration of pigment cells

RA inhibits the migration of B16 murine melanoma cells in vitro, when assayed on polycarbonate membranes or on type I collagen. Using a reconstituted basement membrane invasion assay, in vitro all-*trans*-RA has been shown to bring about dose- and time-dependent inhibition of the ability of A375 human melanoma cell lines to penetrate Matrigel-coated filters.

In RA-treated B16 cells, changes in the cytoskeleton have been observed. This suggested that these RA-induced modifications in the microtubule and microfilament system could be responsible for the inhibition of migration. Treated cells were conspicuously flattened and also appeared to be more adherent to the substrate than untreated cells. Changes in shape of the pigment cells may account for their increased cell adhesion and thus for decreased migration.

In A375 human melanoma sublines, the inhibitory effect of RA on tumour cell invasion was related to a decreased secretion of collagenolytic enzymes with a decrease in the level of type IV collagenase mRNA, to a decreased tissue plasminogen activator, to an increase in the high-affinity metastasis-associated cell surface laminin receptor and to decreased expression of a cell surface receptor for motility factor.[63] Although these results are more closely related to tumour biology, they demonstrate that RA is able to alter cytoskeletal proteins and cell surface receptors of malignant pigment cells. It is most likely that changes of these various molecules also occur on normal human melanocytes. A recent study reports that RA treatment of normal human melanocytes grown in serum-free culture medium alters their morphological appearance. Alterations included retraction of dendritic processes and increased flattening. Studies in these fields are certainly needed as interaction of RA with these different classes of molecules could partly explain some of the clinical effects of RA on melanocytes in vivo.

Nuclear retinoic acid receptors, retinoid-binding proteins and vitamin A metabolism in pigment cells

RA and its derivatives are thought to elicit their physiological effects by binding to nuclear retinoic acid receptors. Two families of nuclear receptors, retinoic acid (RARs) and retinoid X (RXRs) receptors have been identified. In S91 melanoma cells, transcripts complementary to an RAR-γ probe were expressed only at a low level and their expression was unaffected by RA,[64] as was the expression of RAR-α. On the other hand, the induction of RAR-β is dose-dependent, rapid and insensitive to cycloheximide. Both 13-cis-RA and the 3,4-didehydro derivative of RA also induce expression of RAR-γ, but are only effective at a concentration a hundred-fold greater than all-trans-RA.

S91 melanoma cells also constitutively express RAR-α and RAR-γ mRNAs. Similar findings have been obtained in B16 F1 and K-1735P murine melanoma cells. The level of RAR-β mRNA is increased by RA (10^{-7} to 10^{-6}) only in B16 F1 and S91 melanoma cells.[61] The mechanism of this induction is not yet known, but results suggest that binding to cellular retinoic-acid-binding proteins (CRABP) is not required for the modulation of RAR mRNA levels in this system.[61]

RXR-α and -β are also constitutively expressed in B16 melanoma cells, while RXR-γ mRNA levels are not detectable.[65] Long-term retinoic acid treatment decreases the expression of RXR-α but not RXR-β mRNAs.[63] Further experimental data suggest that an unstable transcription factor negatively regulates the expression of RXR-β in these cells. The induction of RXR-β mRNA is direct and occurs within 2 hours after the addition of RA. A recent report[66] demonstrates that normal human epidermal melanocytes in vitro express RAR-α, RAR-β, RAR-γ and RXRa-α, the 9-cis-RA receptor. RAR-γ is the predominant isotype in these cultured cells (personal observations). These four nuclear RA receptors were also detected in four human melanoma cell lines.[64]

Messenger RNA transcripts for the cellular retinol- and retinoic acid-binding proteins (CRBP, CRABP I ands II) are also detected in normal cultured epidermal melanocytes.[66]

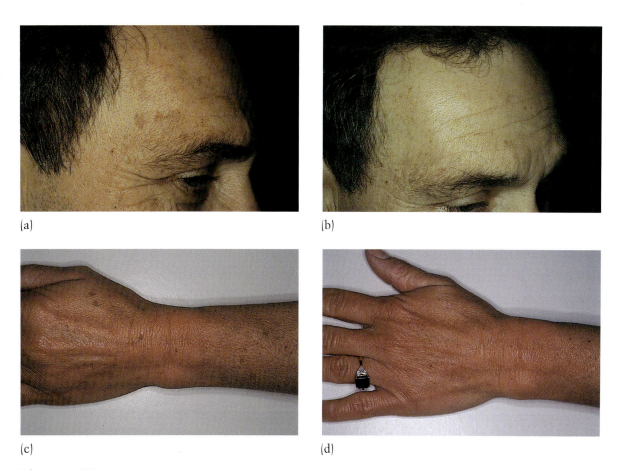

Figure 3.29

Laser treatment (pulsed dye laser 510 nm) of actinic lentigo. (a, c) Before treatment; (b, d) after treatment.

Expression of CRABP I is high in normal melanocytes, whereas CRABP II is the major transcript in human melanoma cells.

This study also demonstrates dissimilarities in the metabolism and endogenous concentrations of retinoids between benign and malignant melanocytes. The endogenous concentrations of retinol and its metabolite 3,4-didehydroretinol in melanocytes were five times those in melanoma cells.

A lack of 9-*cis*-RA formation was also detected in these cells. Furthermore, both melanocytes and melanoma cells produced an unidentified metabolite when incubated with [8^3H]ROH and [^{3}H]RA. The biological significance of the low expression of CRABP I and light expression of RAR-β in melanoma cells compared with melanocytes is unknown.

The effects of RA on pigment cells are multiple and complex. Although the beneficial action of topical RA on pigmentary abnormalities of photoaged skin is well established, the basic mechanisms underlying these effects are not known. Further studies are needed using pure human melanocyte culture as well as mixed keratinocyte–melanocyte culture to evaluate the action of RA on melanogenesis. In vivo studies are also necessary as it is not always possible to extrapolate from in vitro observation to the in vivo situation, particularly in the field of retinoid pharmacology.

Lasers

Most of the 'pigmented' lasers are very efficient at removing actinic and senile lentigines. These lasers include dye (510 nm), copper (511 nm), krypton (520–530 nm), frequency-doubled Q-switched ruby (694 nm) and Q-switched Nd: Yag (1064 nm). All these wavelengths effectively damage pigmented lesions without disrupting the surrounding tissue.

The non-pulsed green light lasers (i.e. krypton, copper, argon), although efficacious in treating superficial epidermal pigmented lesions such as actinic lentigines, do not produce the uniformly good results seen following treatment with the dye (Figure 3.29), frequency-doubled Q-switched ruby, Q-switched Nd:Yag and Alexandrite lasers. In most cases, a single treatment using a low fluence (2.5 J/cm^2) cleans actinic lentigines with minimal side-effects consisting of mild, transient erythema and pigmentary and texture changes. In a few patients, two or three treatments are required to clear the lesions. Pulsed selective therapy using the Q-switched ruby laser or Q-switched Nd:Yag laser may pose less risk of depigmentation or scarring than other techniques, but this remains to be demonstrated.[67]

Laser skin resurfacing is a very promising new treatment for facial rhytides of photoaging. However, postlaser hyperpigmentation is one of the most noted immediate and mid-term side-effects of this therapy. This hyperpigmentation persists for 6–16 weeks. This may be treated with alternating tretinoin and hydroquinone preparations.[68] Laser skin resurfacing can be used in skin phototypes III and IV, provided that pre- and postoperative management is implemented to reduce the risk of dyspigmentation. Patients should use tretinoin, hydroquinone and desonide cream both pre-and postoperatively, along with broad-spectrum suncreens after treatment.

Cryotherapy of actinic lentigo

Melanocytes are particularly susceptible to freezing. Thus cryosurgery is an excellent therapeutic option for the treatment of localized lesions such as actinic lentigines. Liquid nitrogen can be applied by dipping a cotton bud into the flask, or as an open spray from a cryogun or by use of a probe. In most cases, a single treatment (5–10 seconds of freezing) gives a good result.[69] For widespread changes, full-face cryo-peels can be used for effective depth-controlled removal of pigmented lesions.[70] Side-effects limit this treatment approach, however. Prolonged freezing of the skin induces a permanent loss of pigmentation, i.e. an unacceptable cosmetic result. A recent study of the effectiveness of two laser modalities (argon laser light delivered by a Dermascan shuttered delivery system and low-fluence carbon dioxide laser) in comparison with liquid nitrogen cryotherapy concluded that the latter approach is superior in the treatment of lentigines.[71]

Peeling

The α-hydroxy-acids are a class of compounds that are derived from food sources. Glycolic acid, found in sugar cane, is a very useful chemical peeling agent. When glycolic acid is applied on the skin at 50–70% concentrations, many lesions of photoaged skin are improved, including actinic lentigines. For ideal results in the treatment of these lesions, the glycolic acid concentration should be 70% and the solution should be left on the skin for 4–6 minutes.[70] In patients with dark skin, postpeel hyperpigmentation using glycolic acid is a risk, but is less of a risk when using repeated coats of Jessner's solution or 35% trichloroacetic acid.[79] Thus, glycocolic acid peel is regarded as a very good therapeutic strategy for the improvement of pigmentary abnormalities of photoaged skin with minimal risk.

In normal human melanocytes in culture, low doses of ammonium lactate up-regulates cell proliferation, melanogenic protein and tyrosinase activity. In contrast, higher doses of ammonium lactate induce a dramatic down-regulation of melanogenic proteins (tyrosinase and tyrosinase-related protein I). In addition, topical treatment of human skin xenografts on nude mice with ammonium lactate inhibits melanogenic proteins. Interestingly, in this experimental model the expression of a newly identified melanogenic inhibitor present in the human grafts/nude mice was significantly up-regulated by the treatment with ammonium lactate. These results suggest that ammonium lactate has a potential effect on the human pigmentary system.[73]

Application of 25% glycolic acid, lactic acid or citric acid to photoaged skin induces dispersion of melanin pigmentation, in keeping with the clinical improvement of dyspigmentation.[74]

Topical tretinoin before and after a medium-depth chemical peel with 40% trichloracetic acid induces a moderate to marked improvement of lentigines. Although the degree of improvement is significantly higher than in patients with 40% trichloracetic peel alone, the difference is not statistically significant.[75]

Depigmenting agents

A wide range of compounds are recognized as depigmenting agents when topically applied. Skin bleaching or lightening creams are widely advertised. However, very few of them effect clinical improvement. The active constituent of most effective and relatively safe agents for lightening skin pigment is hydroquinone. This chemical inhibits tyrosinase and prevents the conversion of tyrosine to dihydroxyphenylalanine, a precursor of melanin. The maximum concentration of hydroquinone required by regulations is 2% in skin-lightening cosmetic creams. However, at these concentrations, the treatment results are disappointing. Even at a concentration of 5%, hydroquinone creams are reported to be moderately effective in 80 per cent of cases. In order to improve the depigmenting potency of hydroquinone, a formulation associating 5% hydroquinone, 0.1% tretinoin and 0.1% dexamethasone has been used.[76] This formula is therapeutically effective in the treatment of various cutaneous hypermelanoses. However, senile lentigines were resistant to this therapy. Even with three to four applications daily, only slight depigmentation was achieved.

A solution containing 2% 4-hydroxyanisole and 0.01% tretinoin improves solar lentigines. This preparation is significantly superior to each of its components for the treatment of lesions on the face and forearms.[77]

Dermabrasion

Both the superficial dermabrasion with wire brush or diamond fraise produce moderate to marked improvement of lentigines in photoaged skin at 12 weeks after treatment.[76] Histological examination of treated skin demonstrates a significant decrease in the number of epidermal melanocytes. Thus, superficial dermabrasion appears to be efficacious for the treatment of dyspigmentation of photoaged skin. However, the common occurrence of residual hypopigmentation limits the use of this treatment.

References

1. Ortonne JP, Pigmentary changes of the ageing skin. *Br J Dermatol* (1990) **122**: 21–8.
2. Breathnach AS, Nazzaro-Porro M, Passi S, Picardo M, Ultrastructure of melanocytes in chronically sun-exposed skin of elderly subjects. *Pigment Cell Res* (1991) **4**: 71–9.
3. Azizi E, Lusky A, Kushelevsky AP, Schewach-Millet M, Skin type, hair color, and freckles are predictors of decreased minimal erythema ultraviolet radiation dose. *J Am Acad Dermatol* (1988) **19**: 32–8.
4. Valverde P, Healy E, Jackson I et al, Variants of the melanocyte-stimulating hormone receptor gene are associated with red hair and fair skin in humans. *Nat Genet* (1995) **11**: 328–30.
5. Garbe C, Büttner P, Weib J et al, Associated factors in the prevalence of more than 50 common melanocytic nevi, atypical melanocytic nevi and actinic lentigines: multicenter case-control study of the central malignant melanoma resitry of the German Dermatological Society. *J Invest Dermatol* (1994) **102**: 700–5.
6. Nakagawa H, Rhodes AR, Momtaz T-K, Fitzpatrik TB, Morphologic alteration of epidermal melanocytes and melanosome in PUVA lentigines: a comparative ultrastructural investigation of lentigines induced by PUVA and sunlight. *J Invest Dermatol* (1984) **82**: 101–7.
7. Bologna JL, Reticulated black solar lentigo ('ink spot' lentigo). *Arch Dermatol* (1992) **128**: 934–40.
8. Roth DE, Hodge SJ, Callen JP, Possible ultraviolet A-induced lentigines: a side effect of chronic tanning salon usage. *J Am Acad Dermatol* (1989) **20**: 950–4.
9. Salisbury JR, Williams H, du Vivier AWP, Tanning-bed lentigines: ultrastructural and histopathologic features. *J Am Acad Dermatol* (1989) **21**: 689–93.
10. Rhodes AR, Harrist TJ, Momtaz TK, The PUVA-induced pigmented macular: a lnetiginous proliferation of large, sometimes cytologically atypical, melanocytes. *J Am Acad Dermatol* (1983) **9**: 47–58.
11. Maize JC, Ackerman AB, *Pigmented lesions of the skin. Clinicopathologic correlations.* Lea and Febiger: Philadelphia, 1987, pp. 307–11.
12. Leder M, Erythrosis interfollicularis colli. *Dermatologica* (1944) **89**: 132–8.
13. Colomb D, Racouchot J, Gho A, Vernet G, Lerythrosis interfollicularis colli de Leder. *Ann Dermatol Venered* (1997) **104**: 238–42.
14. Borkovic SP, Scwartz RA, McNutt NS, Unilateral erythromelanosis follicularis faciei et colli. *Cutis* (1984) **33**: 163–70.
15. Wheeland RG, Applebaum J, Flashlamp-pumped pulsed dye laser therapy for poikiloderman of Civatte. *J Derm Surg Oncol* (1990) **16**: 12–16.
16. Pope DJ, Sorohan T, Marsden JR et al, Benign pigmented naevi in children. Prevalence and associated factors: the West Midlands, United Kingdom Mole Study. *Arch Dermatol* (1992) **128**: 1201–6.
17. Harrison SL, MacLennan R, Speare R, Wronski I, Sun exposure and melanocytic naevi in young Australian children. *Lancet* (1994) **344**: 1529–32.
18. Cohen LM, Lentigo maligna and lentigo maligna melanoma. *J Am Acad Dermatol* (1995) **33**: 923–36.
19. Gaspar ZS, Dawber RPR, Treatment of lentigo maligna. *Austral J Dermatol* (1995) **61**: 223–47.
20. National Institutes of Health Consensus Development Conference Statement on Diagnosis and Treatment of Early Melanoma, January 27–29, 1992. *Am J Dermatopath* (1993) **15**: 34–43.
21. Elwood JM, Melanoma and ultraviolet radiation. *Clinics Dermatol* (1992) **10**: 41–50.
22. Armstrong BK, Kricker A, English DR, Sun exposure and skin cancer. *Australas J Dermatol* (1997) **58**: S1–S6.
23. Swetter SM, Malignant melanoma from the dermatologic perspective. *Surg Clin North Am* (1996) **76**: 1287–98.
24. Rosso S, MacKie R, Zanetti R, Sun exposure UVA lamps and risk of skin cancer: epidemiological studies. *Eur J Cancer* (1994) **30A**: 548–60.
25. Ortonne JP, Mosher DB, Fitzpatrick TB, *Vitiligo and Other Hypomelanosis of Hair and Skin.* Monograph in Topics in Dermatology. Plenum: New York, 1983.
26. Ortonne JP, Perrot H, Idiopathic guttate hypomelanosis. *Arch Dermatol* (1980) **116**: 664–8.

27. Morison WL, Kerker BJ, Tunnessen WW, Farmer ER, Disseminated hypopigmented keratoses. *Arch Dermatol* (1991) **127**: 848–50.
28. Falabella R, Escobar G, Giraldo N et al, On the pathogenesis of idiopathic guttate hypomelanosis. *J Am Acad Dermatol* (1987) **16**: 35–44.
29. Ploysangam T, Dee-Ananlap S, Suvanprakorn P, Treatment of idopathic guttate hypomelanosis with liquid nitrogen: light and electron microscopic studies. *J Am Acad Dermatol* (1990) **23**: 681–4.
30. Colomb D, Stellate spontaneous pseudoscars. *Arch Dermatol* (1972) **105**: 551–4.
31. Quevedo WC, Szabo G, Virks J, Influence of age and UV on the population of dopa-positive melanocytes in human skin. *J Invest Dermatol* (1969) **52**: 287–90.
32. Gilchrist BA, Blog FB, Szabo G, Effects of ageing and chronic sun-exposure on melanocytes in human skin. *J Invest Dermatol* (1979) **73**: 77–83.
33. Stegmaier OC, Natural regression of the melanocytic nevus. *J Invest Dermatol* (1959) **32**: 413–19.
34. Yeatman JM, Marks R, Kilkenny M, The prevalence of seborrhoeic keratoses in an Australian population: does exposure to sunlight play a part in their frequency? *Br J Dermatol* (1997) **137**: 411–14.
35. Teraki E, Tajima S, Manaka I et al, Role of endothelin-1 in hyperpigmentation in seborrhoeic keratosis. *Br J Dermatol* (1996) **135**: 918–23.
36. Nanninga PB, Ghanem GE, Lejeune FJ et al, Evidence for alpha-MSH binding sites on human scalp hair follicles: preliminary results. *Pigment Cell Res* (1991) **4**: 193–8.
37. Johnson R, Jackson IJ, Light is a dominant mouse mutation resulting in premature cell death. *Nat Genet* (1992) **1**: 226–9.
38. Veis DJ, Sorenson CM, Shutter JR, Korsmeyer SJ, Bcl-2 deficient mice demonstrate fulminant lymphoid apoptosis, polycystic kidneys, and hypopigmented hair. *Cell* (1993) **75**: 229–40.
39. Barker D, Dixon K, Medrano EE et al, Comparison of the responses of human melanocytes with different melanin contents to ultraviolet B irradiation. *Cancer Res* (1995) **55**: 4041–6.
40. Halaban R, Langdon R, Birchall N et al, Basic fibroblast growth from human keratinocytes is a natural mitogen for melanocytes. *J Cell Biol* (1988) **107**: 1611–19.
41. Yada Y, Higuchi K, Imokawa G, Effects of endothelins on signal transduction and proliferation in human melanocytes. *J Biol Chem* (1991) **266**: 18352–7.
42. Gilchrist BA, Park HY, Eller MS, Yarr M, Mechanisms of ultraviolet light. Induced pigmentation. *Photochem Photobiol* (1996) **63**: 1–10.
43. Medrano EE, Farooqui JZ, Boissy RE et al, Chronic growth stimulation of human adult melanocytes by inflammatory mediators in vitro: implications for nevus formation and initial steps in melanocyte oncogenesis. *Proc Natl Acad Sci USA* (1993) **90**: 1790–4.
44. Dooley TP, Recent advances in cutaneous melanoma oncogenesis research. *Oncol Res* (1994) **6**: 1–9.
45. Weiss JS, Ellis CN, Headington JT et al, Topical tretinoin improves photoaged skin: a double-blind vehicle-controlled study. *JAMA* (1988) **259**: 527–32.
46. Bhawan J, Gonzalez-Serva A, Nehal K et al, Effects of tretinoin on photodamaged skin. *Arch Dermatol* (1991) **127**: 666–72.
47. Rafal S, Griffiths CE, Ditre CM et al, Topical retinoic acid improves the irregular hyperpigmentation (liver spots) associated with photoaging. *N Engl J Med* (1992) **326**: 368–74.
48. Goh JH, The treatment of visible signs of senescence: the Asian experience. *Br J Dermatol* (1990) **122**: 105–9.
49. Griffiths CEM, Goldfarb MT, Finkel LJ et al, Topical tretinoin (retinoic acid) treatment of hyperpigmented lesions associated with photoaging in Chinese and Japanese patients: a vehicle-controlled trial. *J Am Acad Dermatol* (1994) **30**: 76–84.
50. Kotrajaras R, Kligman AM, The effect of topical tretinoin on photodamaged facial skin: the Thai experience. *Br J Dermatol* (1993) **129**: 302–9.
51. Uno H, Cappas A, Dong S, Kligman AM, The effect of topical tretinoin on the facial pigmented spots of the stump-tailed macaque. *Eur J Dermatol* (1994) **4**: 471–5.
52. Zheng P, Kligman AM, Topical tretinoin stimulates melanogenesis in the Yucatan micropig. *J Invest Dermatol* (Abstract) (1991) **96**: 576.
53. Edwards L, Jaffe P, The effect of topical tretinoin on dysplastic nevi. *Arch Dermatol* (1990) **126**: 494–9.

54. Ortonne JP, Retinoic acid and pigment cells: a review of in-vitro and in-vivo studies. *Br J Dermatol* (1992) **127**: 43–7.
55. Lotan R, Lotan D, Enhancement of melanotic expression in cultured mouse melanoma cells by retinoids. *J Cell Physiol* (1981) **106**: 179–89.
56. Orlow S, Chakraborty A, Boissy R, Pawelek J, Retinoic acid and other inducers of tumor cell differentiation inhibit the induction of pigmentation in Cloudman melanoma cells. *J Invest Dermatol* (1991) **94**: 562.
57. Yarr M, Gilchrist BA, Human melanocyte growth and differentiation: a decade of new data. *J Invest Dermatol* (1991) **97**: 611–17.
58. Roméro C, Aberdam E, Larnier C, Ortonne J-P, Retinoic acid as modulator of UVB-induced melanocyte differentiation. Involvement of the melanogenic enzymes expression. *J Cell Sci* (1994) **107**: 1095–1103.
59. Ho KKL, Halliday GM, Barnetson RSC, Topical retinoic acid augments ultraviolet light-induced melanogenesis. *Melanoma Res* (1992) **2**: 41–5.
60. Talwar HS, Griffiths CEM, Fisher GJ et al, Topic retinoic acid induces tyrosinase activity in skin of white individuals in vivo. *J Invest Dermatol* (Abstract) (1992) **98**: 645.
61. Clifford JL, Petkovich M, Chambron P, Lotan R, Modulation by retinoids of mRNA levels for nuclear retinoic acid receptors in murine melanoma cells. *Mol Endocrinol* (1990) **4**: 1546–55.
62. Niles RM, Lowey B, B16 mouse melanoma cells selected for resistance to cyclic AMP-mediated growth inhibition are cross-resistant to reinoic acid-induced growth inhibition. *J Cell Physiol* (1991) **147**: 176–81.
63. Hendrix MJC, Wood WR, Seftor EA et al, Retinoic acid Acid inhibition of human melanoma cell invasion through a reconstituted basement membrane and its relation to decreases in the expression of proteolytic enzymes and motility factor receptor. *Cancer Res* (1990) **50**: 4121–30.
64. Latham JAE, Daly A, Todd C et al, Retinoic acid receptor expression in Sg1 melanoma cells: stable induction of RAR-β in response to retinoic acid. *J Invest Dermatol* (1990) **95**: 478.
65. Desai DS, Niles RM, Expression and regulation of retinoid X receptors in B16 melanoma cells. *J Cell Physiol* (1995) **165**: 349–57.
66. Rosdahl I, Andersson E, Kagedal B, Körma H, Vitamin A metabolism and mRNA expression of retinoid-binding protein and receptor genes in human epidermal melanocytes and melanoma cells. *Melanoma Res* (1997) **7**: 267–74.
67. Taylor CR, Anderson RR, Treatment of benign pigmented epidermal lesions by Q-switched ruby laser. *Int J Dermatol* (1993) **32**: 908–12.
68. Lowe NJ, Lask Griffin ME, Laser skin resurfacing. Pre- and post-treatment guidelines. *Dermatol Surg* (1995) **21**: 1017–19.
69. Sinclair RD, Tzermias C, Dawber R, Cosmetic cryosurgery. In: Baran R, Maibach H (eds) *Cosmetic Dermatology*. Martin Dunitz/Waverly Company: 1994, pp. 541–50.
70. Chicarello SE, Full-face cryo-(liquid nitrogen) peel. *J Derm Surg Oncol* (1992) **18**: 329–32.
71. Stern RS, Dover JS, Levin JA, Arndt KA, Laser therapy versus cryotherapy of lentigines: a comparative trial. *J Am Acad Dermatol* (1994) **30**: 985–7.
72. Moy LS, Murad H, Moy RL, Glycolic acid peels for the treatment of wrinkles and photoaging. *J Derm Surg Oncol* (1993) **19**: 243–6.
73. Zhao H, Kobb E, Zhao Y et al, Studies on the effects of ammonium lactate lotion on human pigmentary system. (Abstract) American Academy of Dermatology Meeting, San Francisco, 1997.
74. Ditre DS, Griffin TD, Murphy GF et al, Effects of α-hydroxy acids on photoaged skin: a pilot clinical, histologic, and ultrastructural study. *J Am Acad Dermatol* (1996) **34**: 187–95.
75. Humphreys TR, Werth V, Dzubow L, Kligman A, Treatment of photodamaged skin with trichloroacetic acid and topical tretinoin. *J Am Acad Dermatol* (1996) **34**: 638–44.
76. Kligman AM, Willis I, A new formula for depigmenting human skin. *Arch Dermatol* (1975) **111**: 40–8.
77. Colby SL, Schwartzel EH, Highton A, Epinette WW, Efficacy and safety of BMS181158/181159 solution (2% 4-hydroxyanisole/0.01% tretinoin) versus individual active agents, and vehicle in the treatment of solar lentigines and related hyperpigmented lesions. (Abstract) American Academy of Dermatology Meeting, San Francisco, 1997.
78. Nelson BR, Metz RD, Majmudar G et al, A comparison of wire brush and diamond fraise superficial dermabrasion for photoaged skin. A clinical, immunohistologic, and biochemical study. *J Am Acad Dermatol* (1996) **34**: 235–43.

4 Photodysplasia and non-melanoma skin cancer

Introduction

Chronic exposure to solar ultraviolet irradiation (UVR) causes damage to the nuclear DNA of epidermal cells and a series of other alterations that may lead eventually to squamous cell cancer (SCC). This march of events is dose-dependent, and although all parts of the exposed skin are involved, the final steps in the process are only evident focally and apparently at random over the exposed skin surface.

In this chapter we will cover epidemiological considerations of non-melanoma skin cancer (NMSC), the clinical consequences of chronic UVR exposure leading eventually to NMSC and the pathological alterations found when such lesions are biopsied. We will also briefly review what is known of the process of UVR-induced NMSC (photocarcinogenesis) and briefly discuss the various treatment options.

The effects of chronic UVR exposure and photocarcinogenesis

Acute exposure to 'sunburn doses' of UVR results in oedema and partial necrosis of the epidermis, and in the subsequent 2–4 days there is increased mitotic activity in this tissue. The epidermal changes in chronically sun-exposed skin are less dramatic morphologically, but of great potential importance functionally. Occasional swollen eosinophilic cells with amorphous homogenized cytoplasm, known as sunburn cells or 'Lichtzellen', may appear scattered in the upper epidermis and are dependent on the degree of recent sun exposure, and irregular thickening of the epidermis is seen, but there is no other visibly apparent sign of damage to nuclear DNA.

Solar UVR as a carcinogen

There can be little doubt that the bulk of NMSC is due to exposure to solar UVR. The incidence of SCC increases with proximity to the equator—it doubles with each 10° decrease in latitude. NMSC occurs on the most light-exposed areas—face, forearms and backs of hands—and mostly afflicts the light-complexioned, least-pigmented individuals. Furthermore, the greater the degree of clinical photodamage, the more the likelihood of solar keratoses and NMSC. If further evidence is needed there are numerous studies with small mammals that confirm that UVB, in particular, is carcinogenic – not to mention the unintentional experiment of psoralen plus

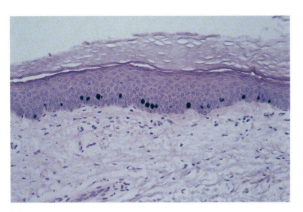

Figure 4.1

Photomicrograph to show thickened epidermis in photodamaged skin. Note that there are many autoradiographically labelled basal epidermal cells after exposure to ^{3}H Thymidine indicating an increased rate of epidermal cell production (haematoxylin–eosin × 45).

ultraviolet A (PUVA) in which UVA is the radiative stimulus and the response is greatly increased rates of development of NMSC (see later).

The 'action spectrum' for carcinogenesis is not known and seems likely to include several wavelengths in the UVB range. Longer wavelengths in the UVA range may also have some carcinogenic potential, or at least a facilitating effect.

Chronic solar injury certainly appears to cause mild to moderate epidermal hypertrophy with irregular epidermal thickening and hypergranulosis (Figure 4.1).[1] There is also slight hyperkeratosis and an increased number of melanocytes in exposed skin. The dose–effect relationship is not well established and it is not known after what dose of UVR chronic changes in the epidermis start to develop, but it may be assumed that individual susceptibility will at least in part determine the time and extent of the response. Although epidermal thickening is usually observed in skin that has been extensively and severely damaged by UVR, epidermal atrophy may occur in a few cases as an end stage to the process. Alongside the epidermal thickening usually seen there are marked histochemical alterations.[2] In particular there is a disproportionate increase in the glucose-6-phosphate dehydrogenase (G6PDH) activity in the upper epidermis in chronically light-exposed skin. We have induced the increased G6PDH activity in previously 'non-exposed' buttock skin by repeated UVR exposure in volunteer subjects and have proposed using this as a model of chronic UVR injury[3] even though we are uncertain as to the importance or significance of the change in relation to neoplastic change.

UVR damage to DNA

Irradiation of the skin with UVR damages DNA, but normal epidermal cells contain 'repair enzymes' that excise segments of damaged DNA and insert new bases to restore the original structure.[4] This process is faulty in xeroderma pigmentosum (see later). Some time after a particular (but unknown) cumulated dose of UVR and after the period over which regular epidermal thickening occurs, another type of change becomes evident. At this juncture it is likely that the capacity for repair of epidermal nuclear DNA after repeated UVR damage becomes exhausted and mutations develop. Mutations to the p53 tumour suppressor gene or to other genes with growth-controlling function such as the *ras* gene and other proto-oncogenes, as well as yet others with tumour-suppressing functions,[5,6] may have an important role to play in the development of keratinocytes with neoplastic potential. Another DNA mechanism that may be involved is what is known as microsatellite instability due to replication errors. The short lengths of DNA involved show alterations in repeat length at multiple foci. This is found to occur in colorectal cancer and has also been found in some patients with non-melanoma skin cancer.[7] One other important and fairly recent finding concerning mutations and basal cell cancer must be mentioned. This is of special interest because the system in which the mutations have been found in the tumour suppressor gene—'patched' in patients with the basal cell naevus syndrome (BCNS). The patched gene encodes a transmembrane protein that opposes a signalling protein known as 'hedgehog' which controls cell fate and growth in many tissues. The mutation in BCNS is heritable, but somatic mutations have also been described in the patched gene in sporadic basal cell carcinoma.[8,9] Clearly, DNA mutations and changes in the regulatory growth factors and mediators controlling epidermopoiesis are of major importance in photocarcinogenesis, but alterations in immune responsiveness may also play a significant role.

UVR-induced immunosuppression

There is reduction in both number and function of Langerhan's cells in light-exposed skin.[10,11] This results in diminished antigen presentation and reduction in the ability to mount a delayed hypersensitivity response. There is strong evidence of the decreased ability to become sensitized to a contact allergen in UV-irradiated skin[12] and this may also result in a failure to eliminate mutated neoplastic consequently antigenically foreign keratinocytes. A study by Yoshikawa et al demonstrated that skin cancer patients were much more susceptible to UVR-induced suppression of DNCB sensitization than a normal control group and were rendered immunologically tolerant to the antigen used.[13] It is well known that immunosuppressed transplant and AIDS patients are at a considerably greater risk for the development of NMSCs.[14,15] Other changes take place in chronically UVR-exposed skin that contribute to a marked functional immunosuppression. Liberation of cytokines from irradiated keratinocytes, including tumour necrosis factor-α and certain of the interleukins, contributes to a dampening of the delayed hypersensitivity response by down-regulating the T helper cell subsets. In addition, exposure to UVR appears to influence the proportion of *cis*- to *trans*-urocanic acid within the upper epidermis and it seems that the UV-induced *cis*-isomer has immunosuppressive properties.[16]

The net result of all these effects is that sun damage causes a reduction in the cellular hypersensitivity immune response and this contributes to the carcinogenic effect of sunlight.

Minimal epidermal dysplasia

The relationships between the DNA alterations and the changes in immune function on the one hand and the histological findings and DNA alterations on the other are not well established and more work is required in this area. The earliest morphological changes observed in the epidermis are in loss of the uniformity of cell size, shape and staining reaction in the cells of the basal and malpighian layers. This results in disturbance to the orderly set of events occurring during differentiation and in a loss of polarity (regular and progressive epidermal differentiation), leading eventually to a subtle but characteristic picture of heterogeneity of cellular and nuclear architecture (Figure 4.2). There is also an increase in epidermal mitotic activity as revealed by tritiated thymidine autoradiographic labelling indices,[17] and a few abnormal mitotic figures make their appearance in the more severely exposed samples of skin. When these abnormal appearances are obvious, but not especially prominent or extensive, the term

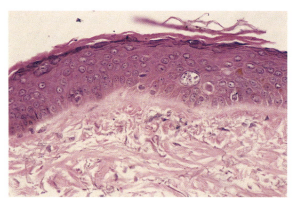

Figure 4.2
Chronically photodamaged skin to show minimal epidermal dysplasia. There is some heterogeneity of cell size and shape and also some dysplastic cells (haematoxylin–eosin ×90).

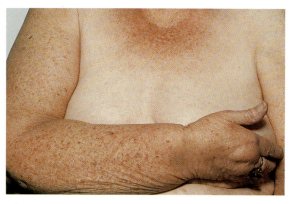

Figure 4.3
Photodamaged skin of forearm held against non-photodamaged upper trunk to show difference between intrinsic aging and photodamage. This type of photodamaged skin often shows minimal epidermal dysplasia.

'minimal dysplastic change' is often used to describe the alteration. Usually it is unaccompanied by parakeratosis or inflammation, which are important discriminatory features of solar keratosis. The term minimal dysplastic change is a histological description without any specific clinical counterpart. The affected skin shows the clinical features of solar elastotic degenerative change (see Chapter 2) and in addition is often irregularly pigmented with dusky hyperpigmentation and senile lentigines focally (see Chapter 3). Apart from these accompanying surface alterations, which are not directly attributable to the underlying epidermal dysplastic change, there may be mild 'drying' of the skin surface with an increased tendency to become slightly scaly if the skin is challenged with chemical, mechanical or climatic stimuli.

Examination of the surface contours of exposed skin by profilometric tracing of skin surface replicas shows that there is gradual effacement of the skin surface markings in the photodamaged areas. This alteration in skin surface markings in exposed sun-damaged skin is not seen on non-exposed skin, which may actually become rougher at some sites.[18]

From the above it seems clear that although there are no specific clinical changes resulting from minimal dysplastic change observed histologically, the battered background clinical appearance of skin is quite characteristic (Figure 4.3) and could justify the suggestion that such an area of skin is likely to show minimal dysplastic changes.

Solar keratosis (syn. actinic keratosis) (SK)

These lesions may be defined as small, discrete, warty and/or inflamed lesions occurring in the sun-damaged skin of elderly subjects that possess a potential for neoplastic change and indicate significant cumulated solar injury.

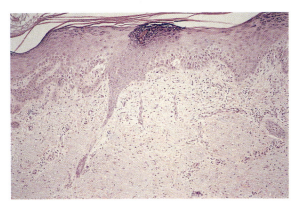

Figure 4.4

Photomicrograph to show Freudenthal's funnel. This is an area of normal epidermal cells surrounded by a minor degree of dysplasia indicating that the eccrine epithelium is unaffected (haematoxylin–eosin ×45).

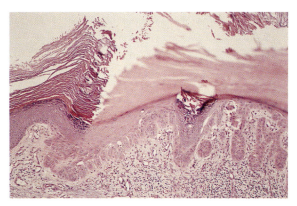

Figure 4.5

Histology of solar keratosis. Note the sloping junction between normal skin and solar keratosis (haematoxylin–eosin ×45).

Histopathology

Characteristically a solar keratosis (SK) will demonstrate areas of marked epidermal dysplasia set against a background of severe solar elastotic degenerative change in the dermis. Because the dysplasia is marked there is usually an accompanying disturbance in epidermal differentiation resulting in parakeratosis. Interestingly, when sweat coils penetrate SKs the eccrine adnexal epithelium is not involved in the surrounding dysplasia, giving rise to a characteristic histological feature in which there is sparing of a segment of the epidermis adjacent to the sweat duct—a feature known as 'Freudenthal's funnel' (Figure 4.4.). The junctions between the abnormal keratinocytes of an SK and the normal epidermis at the margins slope inwards in a rather characteristic manner (Figure 4.5), emphasizing the focal nature of the lesion. The affected epidermis in an SK usually has an irregular dermoepidermal profile and is often thicker than the normal epidermis, although the opposite occurs in

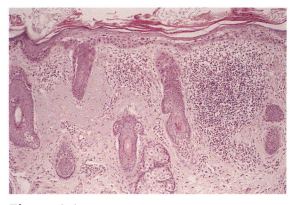

Figure 4.6

Histological section from solar keratosis showing a thin atrophic, but dysplastic epidermis, below which there is considerable inflammation (haematoxylin–eosin ×30).

some instances and then it may be quite thinned (atrophic SK) (Figure 4.6).

Usually there is a variable amount of inflammatory cell infiltrate in the subepider-

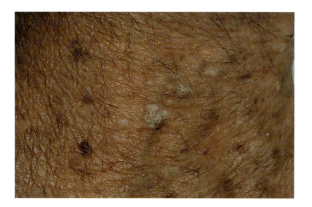

Figure 4.7
Solar keratoses on back of hand.

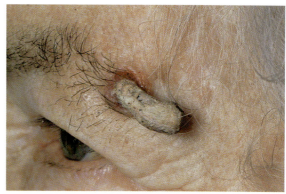

Figure 4.8
Cutaneous horn on side of face.

mal region of an SK. This is for the most part composed of lymphocytes, but there may also be an admixture of plasma cells and histiocytes. In some lesions some of the inflammatory cells find their way into the abnormal epidermis. Immunocytochemical studies have demonstrated that the predominant cell type in the inflammatory cell infiltrate is the T helper lymphocyte subset.[19]

Clinical features and variants

Clinically SKs are for the most part slightly thickened warty or scaling areas approximately 2–10 mm in diameter (Figure 4.7). Sometimes the abnormal horn does not drop off but remains bonded to the surface so that ultimately a 'cutaneous horn' results (Figure 4.8). One common variant of the SK is known as the lupus erythematosus (LE)-like keratosis, which is sometimes confused with a patch of discoid lupus erythematosis (DLE). Both DLE and the so-called LE-like keratosis are characterized by irregular pink scaling and/or hyperkeratotic patches on facial skin (Figure 4.9). Histologically, these LE-like SKs may at times also be embarrassingly difficult to distinguish from DLE as there is often a

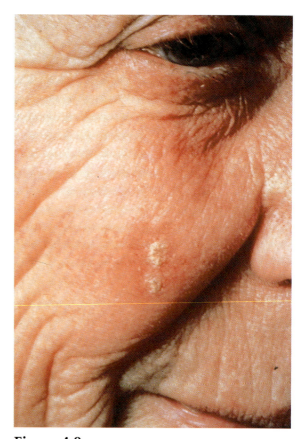

Figure 4.9
Lupus erythematosus-like solar keratosis.

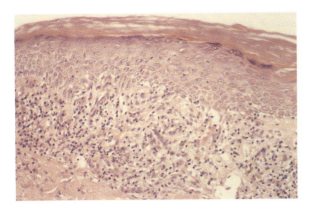

Figure 4.10
Pathology of lupoid lichenoid keratosis showing basal cell erosion and inflammatory cells in the immediate subepidermal zone.

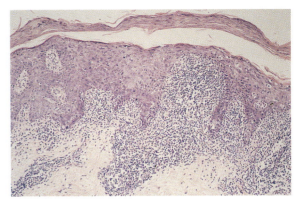

Figure 4.11
Lichenoid solar keratosis. There is a band of inflammatory cells subepidermally.

degree of vacuolar degenerative change in the basal layer (Figure 4.10) in the LE-like keratosis and a marked lymphocytic infiltrate perivascularly in the subepidermal zone.

Some 5–10 per cent of all SKs show basal cell liquefactive degenerative change histologically and in a few this feature may be sufficiently prominent to emulate the condition of lichen planus.[20] In these 'lichenoid SKs' there may also be a 'band-like' subepidermal inflammatory cell infiltrate composed predominantly of lymphocytes (Figure 4.11)— once again compounding the difficulty in confidently making a histological diagnosis. Of course, there is epidermal dysplasia in both the LE-like SK and the lichenoid SK, but this may not be prominent enough to assist in differentiating these variants of SK in every case. It is possible that this lichenoid alteration to SKs indicates that there is 'recognition' by the immune system that the lesion has developed neoantigens which represent a foreign antigenic stimulus and has evoked an attempt at immunological rejection. This mechanism could partially explain why so few SKs progress and many others spontaneously regress (see later). Surprisingly, SKs that show these lichenoid features are indistinguishable clinically from 'ordinary SKs'.[20]

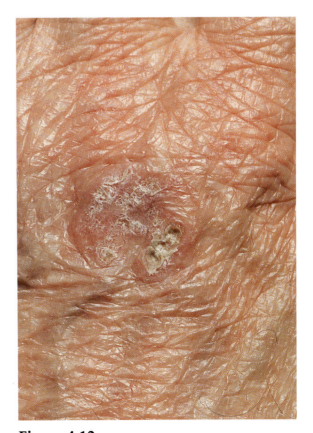

Figure 4.12
Warty slightly pigmented lesion at back of hand which was a solar keratosis histologically.

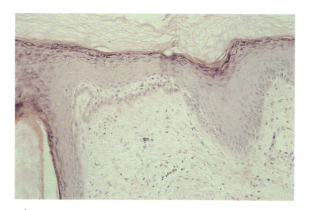

Figure 4.13

Histopathology of acantholytic solar keratosis. There is a band of abnormal cells at the base of the epidermis separated by a slit (haematoxylin–eosin ×90).

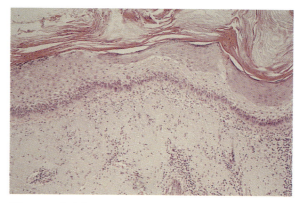

Figure 4.14

Acantholytic solar keratosis. The lower part of the epidermis has an odd spongiotic appearance not uncommonly seen in these lesions (haematoxylin–eosin ×90).

A further clinical variant of SK is a flat, pigmented lesion that is difficult to differentiate from a senile lentigo or a flat seborrhoeic wart.[21] Such pigmented SKs often occur on the temples or the upper cheeks and have only a slightly scaly surface (Figure 4.12). The difficulty in arriving at a firm clinical diagnosis with these pigmented spots is often reflected in their histological picture, which may show features of all of the diagnoses being mooted,[22,23] including senile lentigo, seborrhoeic wart and lentigo maligna.

One further variant of SK is known as the acantholytic solar keratosis (ASK) (this is also known as the Darier-like keratosis and sometimes as carcinoma segregans). It is distinguished by a characteristic histological appearance in which a sheet of dysplastic basal cells appears to have tracked under the basal areas of the neighbouring epidermis and around hair follicles[24,25] (Figure 4.13). The term acantholytic SK stems from the apparent lack of adherence between the abnormal sheet of epidermal cells and the overlying epidermis with the formation of a cleft. Some of the 'migrated' cells become vacuolated, degenerate and spongiotic (Figure 4.14), but whether this change contributes to the cleft formation is unclear. Our study of these lesions could not identify any particular distinctive clinical feature as being associated with the histological features of ASK, although in general, lesions with microscopic characteristics of ASKs appeared larger and more aggressive compared with SKs not showing acantholytic change, as was found in one other previous study.[24]

The biological significance of the ASK is utterly mysterious, but of interest is that it may have relevance to the invasion of tissue by neoplastic cells and the process of metastatic spread. The clinical and histological features of the variants of SK are summarized in Table 4.1.

Prevalence and significance of minimal dysplastic change and solar keratosis

As previously intimated, minimal dysplastic change is frequently present in chronically sun-exposed and photodamaged skin, but because it is not readily clinically separately identifiable, we have very little idea as to the true frequency of this change in the community of what features influence its presence.

Table 4.1 Variants of solar keratosis

Type of SK	Relative frequency	Clinical features	Pathological features
Cutaneous horn	Quite common	Attached hyperkeratotic spiky projection	No special features but marked hypergranulosis and hyperkeratosis
'LE-like' solar keratosis	Quite common	Flat scaling pink patch – mostly on face	Some vacuolar degenerative change in basal layer and sub-epidermal lymphocytic cellular infiltrate common
Lichenoid solar keratosis	5–10% of all lesions sampled show features of lichenoid SK	No typical channge	Vacuolar degenerative change and colloid body formation in basal layer. Marked sub-epidermal inflammation, often very lichen planus (LP)-like
Pigmented solar keratosis	Uncommon	Flat uniformaly pigmented lesion on temple resembling lentigo	Dysplastic change is usually inconspicuous
Acantholytic solar keratosis (syn. Darier-like keratosis – or carcinoma segregans)	Quite common	Tend to be larger and more aggressive	Sheet of dysplastic epithelium appears to be tracking sub-epidermally and round follicles giving appearance of cleft formation.

Perhaps not unexpectedly the epidermis in the clinically uninvolved skin at the sides of SKs demonstrates a marked elevation in mitotic activity.[17] The tritiated thymidine autoradiographic labelling index lies between that for frank lesions of SK and that for unexposed skin of the buttock. The epidermis in chronically sun-exposed sites is thicker and usually shows hypergranulosis and a minor degree of hyperkeratosis. It also shows increased proliferative activity.[1] SKs, on the other hand, are more readily detectable clinically even though clinical accuracy is of the same order as for pigmented lesions.

There have been few studies of the accuracy of the clinical diagnosis of warty skin tumours. It is worth noting that in one recent study the diagnosis of warty lesions was more accurate the longer the dermatologist observing the lesion had been in practice.[26] Overall the accuracy for warty lesions was surprisingly low and certainly not greater then 65–70 per cent.

The work of Robin Marks in a sunny rural part of Queensland, Australia, established that SKs and NMSC were common in the local population. More than 50 per cent of those over the age of 40 had SKs and some 2–3 per cent had SCC.[27] Our own studies in the cool, damp and comparatively sunless South Wales revealed surprisingly that approximately 23 per cent of the population over 60 years of age in South Glamorgan had SKs.[28] The population was sampled according to a randomized and stratified organizational plan. It must be remembered that in the Welsh population there are many who have a Celtic origin and that this ethnic group seems curiously at risk to chronic photodamage of all types.[29] When the populations were surveyed again after a year or longer, a surprisingly large number of lesions had remitted. In the study by Robin Marks and colleagues some 30 per cent of lesions originally noted could no longer be identified. In this study as well as our own it seems that less then one in a thousand SKs transform into SCC.[30] This is a much smaller figure than was originally suggested and it is now clear that the individual SK is not in itself much of a threat. The main implication of the presence of SKs is that the skin has suffered from significant solar damage and in its 'excited state' may develop more aggressive neoplastic lesions somewhere in the exposed area of the skin.

It would be helpful to know more about the UVR stimulus required to generate SKs. For example, how much sun exposure is needed before an SK develops in an outdoor worker? In order to pinpoint the length of time needed the Cardiff group has studied individuals with solar keratoses affecting the bald scalp of elderly men, as it was believed that these individuals would be likely to experience the effects of UVR damage on scalp skin (Figure 4.15). The study suggested that the scalp SKs in our group had appeared some 33 years after the subjects noticed that they were becoming bald.[31]

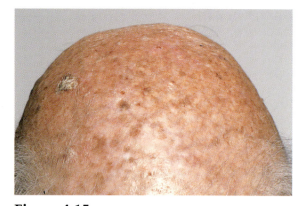

Figure 4.15
Solar keratosis affecting the scalp.

Bowen's disease (syn. intraepidermal epithelioma)

Bowen's disease (BD) can be regarded as the next identifiable milestone along the road to frank malignancy. It is much less common than SK, but appears to arise after significant solar damage in much the same sort of way.

Clinical features

Clinical BD arises on light-exposed and obviously photodamaged skin as one or more red,

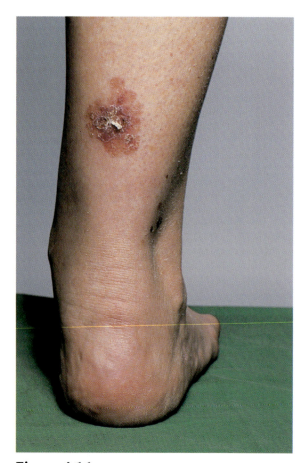

Figure 4.16
Bowen's disease of lower calf in woman.

raised, scaling patches, often with a somewhat psoriasiform appearance. BD lesions tend to be notably thicker than SKs and are usually greater in surface area. A common presentation is a slowly growing psoriasiform scaling plaque on the lower leg in women over the age of 50 (Figure 4.16).[32] Presumably the frequency of these lesions in women is due to the added hazard of both the direct exposure to solar UVR and the reflected UVR from the light-coloured stone of pavements and flooring on to the exposed lower legs below the hemline. Similar lesions occur on the bald scalp of men and the forearms of both sexes.

It has been claimed by some authors that the presence of BD is a marker of a visceral malignancy. Recent studies do not confirm such an association in the great majority of patients.[33] It seems likely that the suggestion arose from patients who had been taking arsenic by mouth for one reason or another (in 'tonics' or in the water supply), as there is a much increased incidence of both visceral and cutaneous cancer in those individuals who have chronically ingested arsenic. Rarely lesions of BD occur in areas that are not obviously exposed to solar UVR. The occasional occurrence of lesions on the fingers or elsewhere on the hands are examples of this. In these sites the lesions may represent neoplastic transformation in a viral wart.[34] Furthermore, lesions analogous to BD occur on the mucosae – as for example erythroplasia of Queyrat on the glans penis, where UVR is clearly not the carcinogen responsible.

Histopathology

The cellular disturbance in BD is similar to that seen in SK save it is more pronounced and effects the entire thickness of the epidermis. There is often a psoriasis-like profile to the epidermal component of the lesion, reflecting the clinical appearance of a psoriasiform plaque. However, the marked dysplasia with bizarre mitotic figures and irregular large cells easily distinguishes the condition from the benign hyperplasia of psoriasis (Figure 4.17). The atypia is sometimes extreme with many bizarre forms and large hyperchromatic irregularly shaped nuclei well deserving of the description *'cellules monstreuses'*. Often there are many abnormal mitoses present as well. There is often a marked degree of inflammation with many lymphocytes subepidermally in typical BD, and just as with SKs the inflammatory cells may be arranged in a 'lichenoid band' and be associated with epidermal basal liquefactive degenerative change. Some of the inflammatory cells cross over into the epidermis. Immunocytochemical studies identify these as T helper lymphocytes.

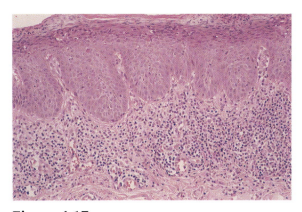

Figure 4.17

Histopathology of Bowen's disease showing irregular psoriasiform thickening and considerable dysplasia.

Disseminated superficial actinic porokeratosis (DSAP)

This order, which was first recognized in the 1960s[35] in the United States, is now believed to be a particular response of the epidermis

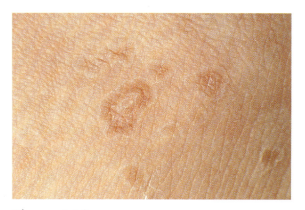

Figure 4.18
Disseminated superficial actinic porokeratosis.

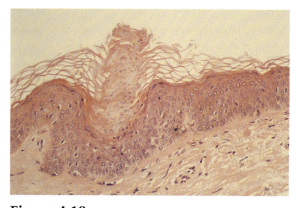

Figure 4.19
Photomicrograph of disseminated superficial actinic porokeratosis showing typical cornoid lamella (haematoxylin–eosin ×45).

on the limbs to persistent solar exposure. Typically the condition occurs in middle-aged women on the front of the lower legs predominantly, but also elsewhere on the limbs (Figure 4.18). The lesions are porokeratosis-like in that they are annular with the slightly raised edge of the lesions containing a narrow horn-filled ridge or vallum (the delicate horny plate in the ridge is known as the cornoid lamella). Histologically, the epidermis shows minimal dysplastic change and a typical parakeratotic horny column (Figure 4.19) in one small, easily missed focal plane. There is also marked lymphocytic reaction in the dermis and vacuolar changes in the basal layer, giving a lichenoid appearance. The findings suggest that DSAP represents a migrating clone of abnormal keratinocytes with an associated immunological host response.[36] Other types of porokeratotic lesion appear to have the propensity for neoplastic change, including naevoid porokeratosis and porokeratosis of Mibelli. Although there do not appear to be reports of SCC occurring in DSAP it would not be surprising if cases were to occur.

Keratoacanthoma (KA) (syn. molluscum sebaceum) and self-healing epithelioma

The KA is a clinicopathological curiosity. It has all the hallmarks of a rapidly growing neoplasm, but regresses just when it looks most threatening.

Clinical features

The usual story obtained from the patient is that the lesion started suddenly as a 'pimple' which then rapidly grew in size. After a rapid growth phase lasting several weeks the increase in size ceases and the lesion is static for some weeks. After a variable period, but mostly 3–6 months, it starts to decrease in size. Ultimately the horny nodule disappears leaving an 'untidy scar'.

Most lesions of KA occur on the face, hands or forearms but a few do develop on non-sun-exposed sites. Most do *not* exceed 1 cm in diameter but uncommonly larger sizes are reached. Typically they take the form of a symmetrical horny nodule with steep walls with a central crater filled with horny debris (Figure 4.20). They often resemble SCC and regrettably there is no certain way of differentiating them clinically. Growth in size continuing unabated after 12 weeks, loss of symmetry and ulceration are amongst the features that should raise the alert that perhaps the lesion is not as benign as was originally believed.

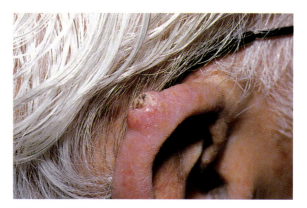

Figure 4.20
Typical keratoacanthoma showing central keratinous plug.

Histopathology

There is a symmetrical area of epidermal thickening in which there is a central horn-filled crypt or invagination. The 'invaginated' area of epidermis is usually partially above the level of the epidermis and partially in the dermis (Figure 4.21). The abnormal epidermis is for the most part bland and unremarkable, showing only a very minor degree of dysplasia, although there may be individual cell keratinization (dyskeratosis). In addition, there is often an irregular border to the basal layer of the cup. Despite the lack of the characteristic features of frank neoplasia it is often difficult to distinguish keratoacanthoma from a well-differentiated SCC and in some cases the ultimate determinant of the nature of the lesion has to be the lesion's clinical behaviour.

Self-healing epithelioma of Ferguson Smith

This lesion is only included here because of its biological similarity to the KA. It is not suspected that it is due to chronic exposure to UVR. It appears to be familial, but its exact mode of inheritance is uncertain. The areas of epidermal thickening form irregular sinuses

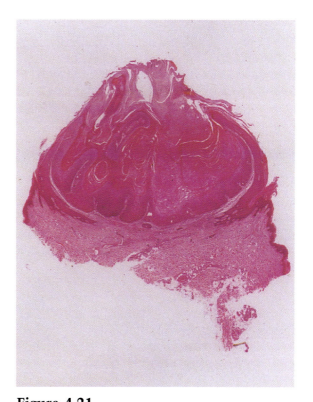

Figure 4.21
Photomicrograph of keratoacanthoma showing horny plug invaginated into an epithelial cup (haematoxylin–eosin ×3).

in the upper parts of the skin and simulate squamous cell epithelioma. Its natural history is much more prolonged than that of the ordinary KA.

Squamous cell carcinoma (SCC) (syn. squamous cell epithelioma)

SCC is the final step towards malignancy, resulting from persistent exposure to solar UVR in the great majority of instances. Solar UVR, however, is not the sole agent responsible for the development of SCC. Chronic heat injury (infrared), X-rays, chemical carcinogens (e.g. dimethyl-benzanthracene experimentally or arsenic in man), some antigenic strains of the human papillomavirus in animals (e.g. HPV 16 and 18) and genodermatoses are other stimuli and factors responsible for the generation of SCCs in some patients.

Clinical features

In most cases the lesions of SCC occur on the exposed skin, but when due to infrared injury often occur on the lower legs. When X-rays or one of the other above-mentioned agents are responsible the resultant SCC can occur anywhere on the skin surface.

SCC lesions usually start off as warty nodules or plaques (Figure 4.22). Occasionally a cutaneous horn is the initial lesion. Later the lesion ulcerates and develops the typical rolled everted edge (Figure 4.23). On the lips infiltrated scaling plaques become fissured and then ulcerate.

Generally the rate of growth of SCC is slow and these lesions do not pose a major threat to life. For the most part metastases are late to develop from SCCs of the limb and trunk skin. SCCs on the lips and ears have a some-

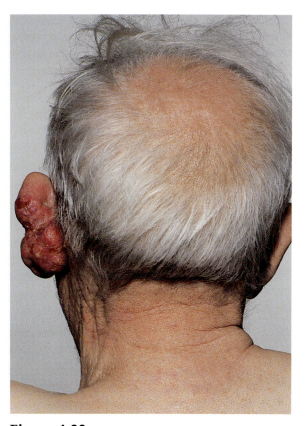

Figure 4.22

Squamous cell carcinoma affecting the left external ear in an elderly man.

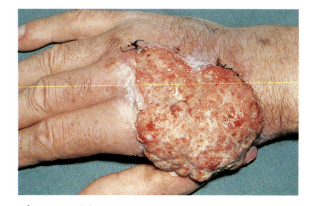

Figure 4.23

Large ulcerated squamous cell carcinoma on back of hand.

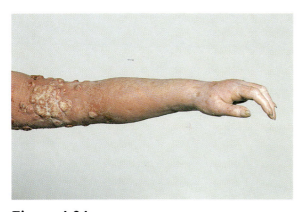

Figure 4.24

Squamous cell carcinoma of the arm with many metastases.

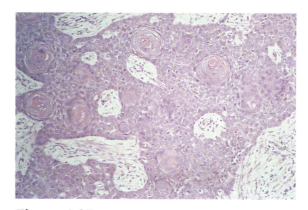

Figure 4.25

Photomicrograph of squamous cell carcinoma showing epithelial masses with fossae of keratinization (horn pearls) and some dysplasia.

what worse reputation. Overall the proportion of SCCs that metastasize appears to be in the order of 5 per cent, but an average figure is almost meaningless. The reason for this is that the term embraces relatively benign lesions that only gradually enlarge and invade locally and quite aggressive cancers that suddenly arise, enlarge and metastasize without warning. Figure 4.24 shows lesions due to local metastatic spread on the arm in a 55-year-old woman who later died as a result of her disease. SCC metastases spread to skin, lungs, bones and brain.

One of the most convincing arguments that UVR exposure causes skin cancer is the increased incidence of NMSC in patients who have been treated with PUVA for psoriasis. Stern and his colleagues from Boston have reported that there is a much greater incidence of SCC in patients with psoriasis treated with PUVA. The incidence of SCC in these patients seems linearly related to the cumulated dose of UVA that they received and the length of time for which they were observed.[37,38] Others have reported a much lesser risk from such UVR treatment and suggested that there is a group at especially high risk who have received other predisposing treatments.[39,40] It should be noted that the male external genitalia seem specially at risk and this region must be carefully shielded to prevent the development of NMSC.[41]

Pathology

The abnormal epithelium is both attached to the superficial epidermis and separated from it as clumps of tumour cells within the dermis. The cells of an SCC vary in their degree of dysplasia with some heterogeneity of cell size, shape and staining reactions as well as nuclear irregularities and loss of polarity. Attempts at keratinization focally result in the formation of rounded masses of horn (horn pearls)—a characteristic feature of SCC (Figure 4.25). The degree of invasiveness is often difficult to determine from a single histological section and many 'step sections' should be studied. It is also difficult to distinguish pseudoepitheliomatous hyperplasia such as is seen for example in nodular prurigo or hypertrophic lichen planus from true but 'low grade' SCC. There are no substitutes for experience and care when it comes to distinguishing the two conditions histologically.

Basal cell carcinoma

Basal cell carcinoma (BCC) is known colloquially as rodent ulcer because in the bad old days when patients sought medical care late in the course of the disease, BCCs progressed to large ulcerated areas which were likened to rat bites. BCCs are said to be the commonest form of human cancer and certainly are an extremely frequent problem in outpatient departments. For example, those consulting with BCC form approximately 3.5 per cent of all new patients in Cardiff. The incidence of BCC is rising in the UK,[42] in the USA, Australia and almost certainly in other affluent, predominantly white Caucasian societies. Although this is almost certainly related to the increasing annual dose of UVR received by the populations concerned, some 10–20 per cent of all BCCs occur on non-exposed skin sites. An unknown proportion of BCCs arise in congenital naevoid disorder or haemartomas such as naevus sebaceous of Jadassohn or other types of

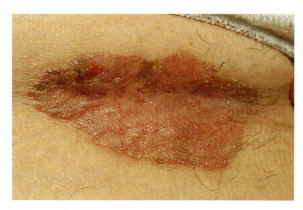

Figure 4.26

Large superficial basal cell carcinoma on trunk.

epidermal naevus. Curiously, superficial BCCs (such as seen in Figure 4.26) occur almost exclusively on non-exposed areas of the trunk.

Clinical types

Nodulocystic

This is the commonest type of BCC. Pearly white or pink opalescent nodular lesions, often

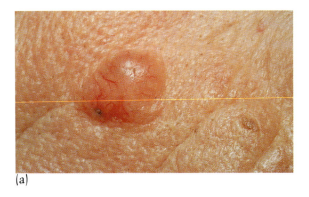

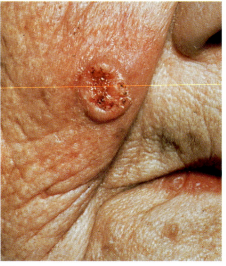

Figure 4.27

(a) Nodular cystic basal cell carcinoma on forehead; (b) ulcerated nodular basal cell carcinoma.

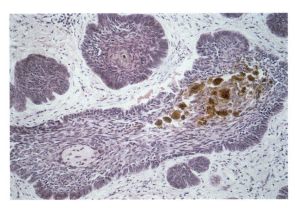

Figure 4.28

Photomicrograph of basal cell carcinoma. This biopsy was taken from a pigmented basal cell carcinoma and large amounts of melanin can be seen within the clumps of basaloid epithelium (haematoxylin–eosin ×45).

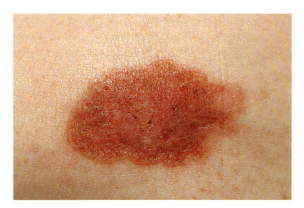

Figure 4.29

Superficial basal cell carcinoma of the trunk.

with telangiectatic vessels coursing over their surface, slowly increase in size over several months or a few years. Ultimately they become eroded, leaving ulcers with raised everted edges (Figure 4.27a, b). They rarely metastasize, although they are capable of doing so,[43] but are always locally destructive and invade surrounding tissues. If they invade cartilage and/or bone they can produce terrible facial deformities if left untreated for long periods.

Pigmented

Not uncommonly, flecks of brown/black pigmentation discolour nodulocystic BCCs, but sometimes this is the predominating clinical feature so that they can be mistaken for naevi or even melanoma (Figure 4.28). Pigmented BCCs are the most frequent type of BCC seen in the basal cell naevus syndrome.

Superficial

This type of lesion may resemble a plaque of psoriasis, a patch of discoid eczema or a lesion of Bowen's disease, but usually has a distinctive thin 'hair-like margin' (Figure 4.29). Superficial BCCs occur almost exclusively on the trunk and may be unassociated with photodamage. They can cover a large area and lesions that cover 5 cm^2 are not particularly uncommon.

Morphoeic

BCCs can provoke a sclerosing fibrotic reaction so that they resemble patches of scleroderma or morphoea both clinically and histologically (Figure 4.30). These lesions are uncommon, but are amongst the most dangerous on account of their atypical appearance, which means that the correct diagnosis is not made at a time when complete removal is comparatively simple. Compounding the difficulty in diagnosis clinically is a similar situation histologically, as there are sparse columns and sheets of BCC cells tracking between bundles of fibrous tissue and these may not be evident in all sections. The histological picture can resemble ordinary morphoea when the characteristic basaloid

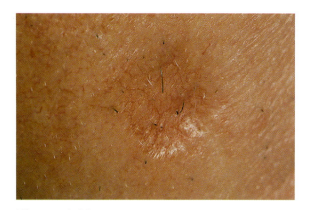

Figure 4.30
Morphoeic basal cell carcinoma. There is some central depression in this pearly plaque.

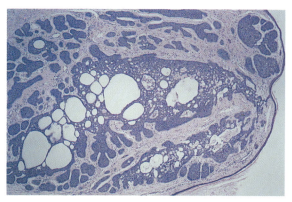

Figure 4.31
Pathology of basal cell carcinoma showing large basaloid clumps of cells in the dermis, many with central degenerative change.

cells are few in number, or when there are small dumps and columns of basaloid cells the disorder can look quite like syringoma.

Pathology of BCC

Typically there are clumps of basaloid cells in the dermis. The clumps vary greatly in size and shape (Figure 4.31). Mostly there is no attempt at differentiation by these cells, but occasionally—especially if they are irritated—there may be foci of vicarious keratinization with small clusters of squamous cells and even horn pearls. On occasion the clumps of abnormal cells appear to emulate pilar or sweat glandular structures in a half-hearted attempt at some form of differentiation towards an adnexal structure. The peripheral cells are often arranged longitudinally to the main mass of cells (an arrangement known as palisading). Degenerative change is often present within the cellular clumps, accounting for the cystic appearance of some lesions. Melanin pigment is often obvious and in some instances is a prominent feature, accounting for the pigmented type of BCC.

In routine paraffin-embedded sections it is common to see a gap between the clumps of BCC cells and the dermal connective tissue. This is known as 'retraction artefact' and is ascribed to the removal of soluble proteoglycan material at the periphery of the cellular masses during fixation and dehydration. The surrounding dermal connective tissue shows a variable amount of inflammation and fibrotic response. In the morphoeic lesion, the fibrotic response is very pronounced and accounts for the clinical features reminiscent of a patch of morphoea.

Other forms of NMSC of uncertain relationship to photodamage

There are large numbers of different carcinomatous lesions originating from sweat and sebaceous glands. Most of these are very uncommon and for the most part are probably not due to solar UVR. These lesions do not appear to have a predilection for sun-exposed skin; although sebaceous gland carcinoma seems to be most frequently found on the nose, this should not be surprising as this site is very rich in these glandular structures compared to other sites. Adnexal epithelium is mostly deep within the skin and out of the direct reach of solar UVR, which does not penetrate very far.

Atypical fibroxanthoma is an odd, rapidly growing, neoplastic disorder which mainly affects the bald scalps of elderly and photodamaged men. Its exact cell of origin is uncertain, but it may be caused or provoked by UVR damage. Although it is rapidly growing and has a histologically bizarre appearance, excision is luckily curative for most patients, but metastatic spread is quite possible.

Merkel cell tumours (syn. trabecular carcinoma) are also very uncommon. They can arise at any body site, although it has been suggested that a UVR exposure does play a role in their development.

Treatment of photodysplasia and non-melanoma skin cancer

Photodysplasia

When there are no focal lesions, but clear evidence of chronic photodamage and histological evidence of minimal epidermal dysplasia, there are good grounds for suggesting therapeutic interventions. Apart from improving the appearance of the photodamaged skin this should reduce the chance of developing keratoses and more definitive forms of NMSC. Reduction in sun exposure will at least stop further damage from occurring and allow repair to take place. The use of sunscreens that protect against both UVB and UVA are also likely to assist in allowing repair to occur. Sunscreen use has certainly been shown to reduce the number of solar keratoses present compared with a control group and in reducing the degree of solar elastosis.[44,45]

Topical tretinoin and isotretinoin have been demonstrated to reduce the signs of photodamage (see Chapter 8) and there is some evidence that they reduce the number of solar keratoses when applied over long periods.[46] These agents probably also reverse minor degrees of epidermal dysplasia, but the data to support this are much more difficult to obtain, involving complicated histological measurements.

The α-hydroxy acids, especially lactic and glycolic acids, have also been reported to improve photodamage, but there is no evidence of reduction in solar keratoses or reduction in photodysplasia after their use.

Peeling the skin with agents such as 70% glycolic acid[47] or laser resurfacing[48] are also effective methods for dealing with photodysplasia and the other changes of photoaging, but are beyond the scope of the present book.

Non-melanoma skin cancer

Surgical excision, curettage or microscopically controlled (Mohs) microsurgery are used, depending on the type and site of the lesion.[49] Radiotherapy is not often used now, but cryotherapy has retained its popularity with some (not shared by the author) for small superficial lesions. The reader is referred to Dawber et al for details as to the surgical techniques mentioned.[50]

References

1. Lavker RM, Cutaneous aging: chronologic versus photoaging. In: Gilchrist BA (ed.) *Photodamage*. Blackwell Science: Cambridge, MA, 1995.

2. Pearse AD, Gaskell SA, Marks R, Epidermal changes in human skin following irradiation with either UVB or UVA. *J Invest Dermatol* (1987) **88**: 83–7.
3. Pearse AD, Marks R, Response of human skin to ultraviolet radiation: Dissociation of erythema and metabolic changes following sunscreen protection. *J Invest Dermatol* (1983) **80**: 191–4.
4. Muramatsu T, Kobayashi N, Tada H et al, Induction and repair of UVB induced cyclobutane pyrimidine dimers and (6-4) photoproducts in organ cultured normal human skin. *Arch Dermatol Res* (1992) **284**: 232–7.
5. Li G, Mitchell DL, Ho VC et al, Decreased DNA repair but normal apoptosis in ultraviolet irradiated skin of p53-transgenic mice. *Am J Path* (1996) **148**: 1113–23.
6. Brash DE, Ziegler A, Jonason AS et al, Sunlight and sunburn in human skin cancer: p. 53, apoptosis and tumour promotion. *J Invest Dermatol* (1996), Symposium Proceedings 1: 136–42.
7. Quinn AG, Healy E, Rehman I et al, Microsatellite instability in human non melanoma skin cancer. *J Invest Dermatol* (1995) **104**: 309–12.
8. Ora AE, Higgins KM, Hu Z et al, Basal cell carcinomas in mice over expressing sonic hedgehog. *Science* (1997) **276**: 817–21.
9. Johnson RL, Rothman AL, Xio J et al, Human homolog of patched, a candidate gene for the basal cell naevus syndrome. *Science* (1996) **272**: 1668–71.
10. Toews GB, Bergstresser PR, Streilein JW, Epidermal Langerhans cell density determines whether contact hypersensitivity or unresponsiveness follows skin painting with DNFB. *J Inmmunol* (1980) **124**: 445–9.
11. Elmets CA, Bergstresser PR, Tigelaar RE et al, Analysis of the mechanism of unresponsiveness produced by haptens painted on skin to low dose UV radiation. *J Exp Med* (1983) **158**: 781–94.
12. Ullrich SE, Modulation of immunity by ultraviolet radiation: Key effects on antigen presentation. *J Invest Dermatol* (1995) **105**: 30S–36S.
13. Yoshikawa T, Rae V, Bruins-Slot W et al, Susceptibility to effects of UVB radiation on induction of contact hypersensitivity as a risk factor for skin cancer in humans. *J Invest Dermatol* (1990) **95**: 530–6.
14. Shuttleworth D, Marks R, Griffin PJ, Salaman JR, Dysplastic epidermal change in immunosuppressed patients with renal transplants. *Quart J Med* (1987) **64**: 609–16.
15. Wang CY, Brodland DG, Su WP, Skin cancers associated with acquired immunodeficiency syndrome. *Mayo Clinic Proceedings* (1995) **70**: 766–72.
16. Gibbs NK, Norval M, Traynor NA et al, Action spectra for the trans to cis photoisomerisation of urocanic acid in vitro and in mouse skin. *Photochem Photobiol* (1993) **57**: 584–90.
17. Pearse AD, Marks R, Actinic keratoses and the epidermis on which they arise. *Br J Dermatol* (1977) **96**: 45–50.
18. Heggie RH, Edwards C, Marks R, The effect of age and sun damage on the roughness of skin. *Br J Dermatol* (1995) **132**: 656.
19. Habets JMW, Tank B, van Joost Th, Characterization of the mononuclear infiltrate in Bowen's disease (squamous cell carcinoma in situ). Evidence for a T cell mediated antitumour immune response. *Virchows Arch A Pathol Anat* (1989) **415**: 125–30.
20. Tan CY, Marks R, Lichenoid solar keratoses: Prevalence and immunological findings. *J Invest Dermatol* (1982) **79**: 365–7.
21. Dinehart SM, Sanchez RL, Spreading pigmented actinic keratosis. *Arch Dermatol* (1988) **124**: 680–3.
22. Rafal ES, Griffiths CEM, Ditre CM et al, Topical tretinoin (retinoic acid) treatment for liver spots associated with photodamage. *N Engl J Med* (1992) **326**: 368–74.
23. Lever LR, Marks R, Pigmented facial macules: a sign of photoaging? In: R Marks, G Plewig (eds) *Acne and Related Disorders*. Martin Dunitz: London, 1992, pp. 91–6.
24. Jablonska S, Chorzelski T, Dyskeratoma and epithelioma (carcinoma) dyskeratoticum segregans. *Dermatologica* (1961) **123**: 24–37.
25. Lever L, Marks R, The significance of the Darier like solar keratosis and acantholytic change in pre-neoplastic lesions of the epidermis. *Br J Dermatol* (1989) **120**: 383–9.
26. Abu-Taha SB, Accuracy of clinical diagnosis of warty lesions. MSc Thesis 1993. University of Wales College of Medicine, Cardiff.
27. Marks R, Ponsford MW, Selwood TS et al, Non melanotic skin cancer and solar keratoses in Victoria. *Med J Austral* (1983) **ii**: 619–22.

28. Harvey I, Frankel S, Marks R et al, Non melanoma skin cancer and solar keratoses I. Methods and descriptive results of the South Wales cancer study. *Br J Cancer* (1996) **74**: 1302–7.
29. Long CC, Marks R, Increased risk of skin cancer: another Celtic myth? A review of Celtic ancestry and other risk factors for malignant melanoma and non melanoma skin cancer. *J Am Acad Dermatol* (1995) **33**: 658–61.
30. Mark R, Rennie G, Selwood TS, Malignant transformation of solar keratoses to squamous cell carcinoma. *Lancet* (1988) **1**: 795–7.
31. Long CC, Turner RJ, Marks R, Actinic keratoses: bald facts. *Arch Dermatol* (1996) **132**: 1132–3.
32. Cox NH, Body site distribution of Bowen's disease. *Br J Dermatol* (1994) **130**: 714–16.
33. Chute CG, Chuang TY, Gergstralh EJ, Su WP, The subsequent risk of internal cancer with Bowen's disease. A population based study. *J Am Med Assoc* (1991) **266**: 816–9.
34. Shuttleworth D, Marks R, Griffin PJA et al, Dysplastic epidermal change in immunosuppressed patients with renal transplants. *Quart J Med* (1987) **243**: 609–16.
35. Chernosky ME, Freeman RG, Disseminated superficial actinic porokeratosis (DSAP). *Arch Dermatol* (1967) **96**: 616–24.
36. Shumack S, Commens C, Kossard S, Disseminated superficial actinic porokeratosis. A histologic view of 61 cases with particular references to lymphocytic inflammation. *Am J Dermatopath* (1991) **13**: 26–31.
37. Stern RS, Lange R, Non melanoma skin cancer occuring in patients treated with PUVA five to ten years after first treatment. *J Invest Dermatol* (1988) **91**: 120–4.
38. Forman AB, Roenigk HH, Caro WA, Long term follow-up of skin cancer in the PUVA – 48 cooperative study. *Am J Dermatopath* (1989) **125**: 515–19.
39. Henselar T, Christophers E, Honigsman H et al, Skin tumours in the European PUVA study. *J Am Acad Dermatol* (1987) **16**: 108–16.
40. Tanew A, Honigsman H, Ortel B et al, Non melanoma skin tumours in long term photochemotherapy treatment of psoriasis. *J Am Acad Dermatol* (1986) **15**: 960–65.
41. De la Brassinne M, Richard B, Genital squamous cell carcinoma after PUVA therapy. *Dermatology* (1992) **185**: 316–18.
42. Koc B, Walton S, Keczkes K et al, The emerging epidermis of skin cancer. *Br J Dermatol* (1994) **130**: 269–72.
43. Von Domarus H, Stevens PJ, Metastatic basal cell carcinoma: report of 5 cases and review of 170 cases in the literature. *J Am Acad Dermatol* (1984) **10**: 1043–60.
44. Naylor MF, Boyd A, Smith DW et al, High sun protection factor sunscreens in the suppression of actinic neoplasia. *Arch Dermatol* (1995) **131**: 170–5.
45. Thompson SC, Jolley D, Marks R, Reduction of solar keratoses by regular sunscreen use. *N Engl J Med* (1993) **329**: 1147–51.
46. Farmer KC, Naylor MF, Sun exposure, sunscreens and skin cancer prevention: a year round concern. *Ann Pharmacother* (1996) **30**: 662–73.
47. Naylor MF, Boyd A, Smith DW, High sun protection factor sunscreens in the suppression of actinic neoplasia. *Arch Dermatol* (1995) **131**: 170–5.
48. Becker FF, Sangfroid FP, Rubin MG, Speelman P, A histological comparison of 50% and 70% glycolic acid peels using solutions with various pHs. *Dermatol Surg* (1996) **22**: 463–5.
49. August PJ, Cryotherapy of non melanoma skin cancer. In: Moy RL, Telfer NR (eds) *Clinics in Dermatology* (1995) **??**: 589–92.
50. Dawber R, Colver G, Jackson A, *Cutaneous Cryosurgery: Principles and Clinical Practice*, 2nd edn. Martin Dunitz: London, 1997.

5 Intrinsic aging of skin

Introduction

Below 10 years it is not usually difficult to guess a child's age from his or her face. After that it becomes increasingly difficult as the years roll by. The reason for this is that we unconsciously relate age to a set of alterations in facial appearance and body habits that are only in part due to the aging process and are mainly the result of accumulated environmentally sustained traumas of different sorts. Prominent amongst these latter are the set of changes that occur in facial skin and are due to the long-continued damaging effect of solar ultraviolet radiation (UVR). These clinical changes are variously referred to as cutaneous photodamage, photoaging, dermatoheliosis and chronic heliodermatitis. All these terms have merits and demerits and it is our prejudice to prefer the use of either photoaging or just 'photodamage' to describe these processes. Other agencies probably add to the accumulated traumata in exposed skin, but these are much less well documented. Cigarette smoking is probably one of these traumas, for there is a growing body of evidence that this habit does indeed lead to or worsen elastotic degenerative change within skin and the clinical appearance of fine lines around the mouth and on the cheeks, though the mechanism is uncertain (Figure 5.1). All tissue alterations resulting from these various external traumas will be superimposed on the process of intrinsic aging. Although intrinsic aging occurs in unexposed skin to the same extent as in exposed skin, it is quite difficult in practice to sort out these inevitable biological alterations from the tissue changes due to photodamage in exposed skin. Another difficulty concerns what is judged to be non-exposed skin. For instance, the volar aspect of the forearm or the inner aspect of the upper arm may, in some subjects, be more sun-damaged than one would imagine.

Intrinsic aging might just as well be called 'inevitable aging' because from what we know

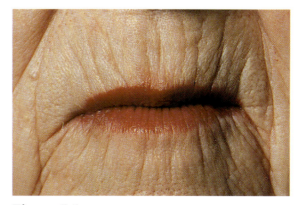

Figure 5.1

Lines around mouth from cigarette smoking.

at present the process is unstoppable, although some of the associated phenomena can be modulated or delayed.[1] As may be expected, aging occurs in all tissues and organs, but it is one of the major mysteries of this process that there is such an enormous variation in the rate of aging in different tissues. Leaving aside the effects of both congenitally determined and acquired disease and trauma of different kinds, individuals display enormous variation in the way they show their years. Some (such as the writer of the Foreword to this book) are physically vigorous and intellectually vibrant into their eighties and others are markedly sagging by their early fifties. The reasons for this diversity, as with so much else about aging, are quite obscure.

There have been concerted efforts to understand the nature of aging, but although some progress has been made and several interesting hypotheses have been advanced, we are a long way off knowing precisely why we age and how this happens. All eukaryotic organisms age and eventually die. The universality of this fundamental characteristic of life surely signifies some essential biological rule which at present eludes us. Is it to do with preserving resources so that the young, newly arrived organisms will have the best chance of surviving? Is the process of aging merely an unfortunate and unstoppable by-product of the complexity of DNA and the biochemistry of life? Mitochondrial DNA may influence longevity. It has recently been reported that particular sequences of DNA were more frequently found in Japanese centenarians than in younger control groups and it was suggested that these special sequences of DNA protected in some way against adult onset degenerative diseases.[2] The length of telomeric DNA also appears to play some role in the aging process. It has been shown that telomeric shortening occurs in explanted primary fibroblasts and this leads to replicative senescence.[3] Telomeric shortening has also been found in blood cells of bone-marrow-transplanted individuals who are well known

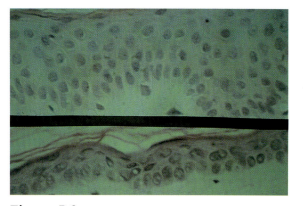

Figure 5.2

Thinned epidermis of old age. The upper section is from a young adult while the lower section is from a man in his 80s. They are both from the abdomen (H. and E. ×90).

to be more likely to develop second leukaemias and other 'clonal' disorders.[4] It was suggested that the replicative stress of repopulating the marrow after transplantation resulted in the telomeric shortening found in the young recipients studied in this report. Biologists have been fascinated by the finding that fibroblasts in culture have a finite ability to multiply,[5] and this phenomenon, known as the 'Hayflick principle', may well be a reflection of the changes in telomeric length.

It has been suggested that the generation of free radicals damages complex macromolecules, which suffer functionally so that they cannot be eliminated and are deposited in the cell causing it eventually to succumb.[6] If this is the main drive to aging than it is really not so different from the biochemical changes caused by environmental traumas.

Epidermal alterations

The epidermis is a sensitive mirror of aging. All elements of the epidermis share in the

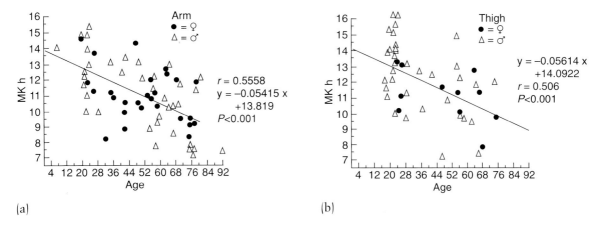

Figure 5.3

Mean keratinocyte height plotted against age for two sites.

attrition of senescence. The whole structure becomes thinner with increasing age, as is evident in histological sections (Figure 5.2). In youth and the mature years, the average number of keratinocytes in the thickness of the epidermis is four or five cells on the trunk or limb skin. At the age of 80 the thickness is reduced to about three cells. Not only is the number of cells reduced, but the size of individual keratinocytes is decreased. Determination of the size of keratinocytes is actually quite a difficult task and the techniques employed are at best compromises between what is technically possible and the ideal realization of true in vivo dimensions. One method used by the author is based on examination of formalin-fixed, paraffin-embedded sections. Projection of the image through the side arm of a microscope and the use of measuring graticules enables figures to be derived for the mean keratinocyte height (Mkh) and mean keratinocyte length (Mkl). In youth and maturity the MKh for the average basal and malphigian keratinocyte is 12 µm and the Mkl is 7.0 µm, giving a mean keratinocyte volume of approximately 600 µm.[7] The value for Mkh was found to decrease gradually with increasing age at the three non-sun-exposed sites investigated—

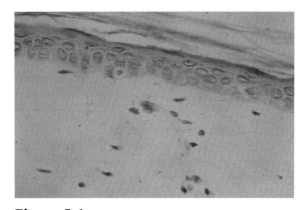

Figure 5.4

Flattening of papillary structure in epidermis from abdomen of man in his 80s (H. and E. ×90).

inner upper arm, outer thigh and lower abdomen (Figure 5.3). Despite the wide variability of the observations it was evident that the Mkh at the age of 80 was only some two-thirds of that at age 20. When checked against frozen histological sections and suspensions of keratinocytes run through a particle counter there was little difference for the values obtained using formalin-fixed and paraffin-embedded tissue by the sample projection technique described.

The overall thinning of the epidermis in old age is accompanied by a reduction in the undulating profile of the epidermis reflecting its papillary arrangement, so that it is altogether a flatter structure (Figure 5.4).

The major function of the epidermis is to produce an efficient structural and diffusional barrier to the outside world—the stratum corneum. Interestingly enough, the altered dimensions of the epidermal structure and its constituent keratinocytes do not seem to be reflected in its stratum corneum end product. In fact, several groups of workers including ourselves have demonstrated that the size of individual corneocytes increases as the individual ages.[7-9] The mean corneocyte area (MCA) at age 20 is approximately 800 μm[6] and at age 80 it is approximately 1000 μm.[6] The paradox of the decreasing size of keratinocytes and the increasing size of corneocytes has not as yet been satisfactorily explained, but may reside in a changed corneocyte thickness—a parameter which currently is extremely difficult to measure accurately.

A further observation which is difficult to explain is the apparent constancy of the thickness of the stratum corneum at all ages. Presumably, a maintained thickness is better able to maintain the vital barrier function necessary for the constancy of the milieu intérieur. Curiously, there are some hints that the stratum corneum barrier is somewhat more efficient in the elderly. This certainly seems to apply as far as transepidermal water loss is concerned and maybe it applies to percutaneous penetration as well.[10] This improved function seems to be the result of there being corneocytes with greater surface area in the stratum corneum of elderly subjects, causing a reduction in intercorneocyte space per unit volume of stratum corneum[11] (Figures 5.5 and 5.6). As transepidermal water loss seems to depend on the intercorneocyte compartment, it is reasonable to attribute the small changes in this function in the elderly to this alteration in

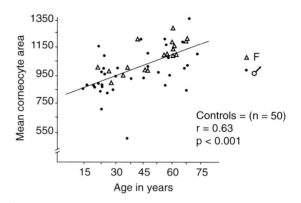

(a)

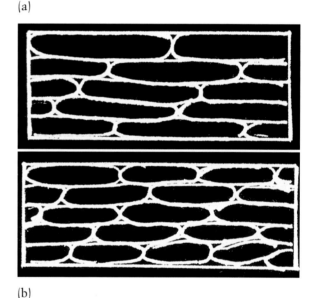

(b)

Figure 5.5

(a) Relationship between corneocyte area and age. (b) Reduction in intercorneocyte space with larger corneocytes. The upper diagram from the strata corneum of an older person with larger corneocytes contains less intercorneocyte space per unit volume.

structural relationships. The same is probably true of the percutaneous penetration of drugs and xenobiotics, but data on this aspect of stratum corneum function are hard to obtain.

The reduced population of epidermal cells in the relatively thin and flat aged epidermis

Intrinsic aging of skin

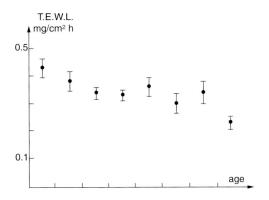

Figure 5.6

Transepidermal water loss decreases as a function of age. (From Tan CY, Stratham B, Marks R et al, Skin thickness measurement by pulsed ultrasound: Its reproducibility, validation and variability. *Br J Dermatol* (1984) **23**: 322–9.)

suggests that the rate of cell production is decreased. There is no doubt that the rate of stratum corneum renewal is decreased in elderly subjects and the turnover time for the structure is lengthened as measured using a dansyl chloride fluorescence extinction time technique.[12] The data for epidermal cell renewal might be expected to parallel the slower turnover time of the stratum corneum, but because of technical considerations, the situation is less clear-cut. Certainly some authors have reported that there is a reduction in the number of cells in DNA synthesis as determined using a tritiated thymidine autoradiographic labelling index method.[13] Observations from the writer's own laboratory have not confirmed this reduction. Other difficult-to-measure factors, including the length of the DNA synthesis phase, the growth fraction and the rate of apoptosis, also influence the keratinocyte pool size, so that the issue is somewhat complicated. At present we cannot say which of these various factors is (or are) responsible for any observed change in replicative activity.

The unexposed skin of the elderly does not usually show dramatic alterations to the naked eye. It may be slightly paler than it had been in youth due to loss of melanin pigment (see later), but the main changes are only evident to the probing finger. There are difficult-to-define subjective surface textural changes detected by the probing finger which are at least in part the result of modification of the skin surface contour. Findings from the author's laboratory suggest that in non-exposed skin, skin surface contour shows some increasing irregularity with increased age.[14] Opposite findings have been reported by other groups.[15] The differences could be due to differences in the techniques employed or perhaps in the interpretation of the data obtained, but whatever else is true it seems intrinsically unlikely that any of the small differences present in surface texture could explain most of the alteration in the feel of the skin of the elderly. Other contributory factors which influence the changed perception include decreased water content of the horny layer in the elderly,[16] decreased rates of sweat[17] and sebum secretion[18] in the elderly and alterations in the structural features of their hair.[19] Many changes occur in the hair of the elderly and only a brief summary can be included here. The rate of growth slows and the length of the growth phase—anagan—decreases, so the hair needs cutting less frequently. The number of follicles per unit area also decreases so that all in all the impression is that the skin is less 'hairy'. Greying of the hair is a function of aging, but it is the most variable of the changes and can occur surprisingly early in life. The above applies to both body and scalp hair, although the alterations are much more noticeable on the scalp. The curious phenomenon known as male pattern alopecia is made more evident by the aging process, but is not part of it.

The nail plates are also altered by age. The fingernails tend to be thinned and longitudinally ridged in old age, but the toenails often develop a quite 'psoriasis-like' appearance,

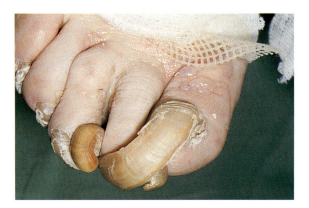

Figure 5.7
Early onychokygryphosis in an elderly woman.

even though there is no hint of psoriasis elsewhere, and may be thickened and yellowed and in a few patients curl up in a most curious way in the condition known as onychokygryphosis. They certainly grow much less rapidly in the elderly.[20] Some speak wistfully of the 'bloom of youth', suggesting some almost mystical quality that the skin possesses in the early years of life which is lost during aging. As yet we have no way of characterizing or quantifying this co-called bloom and can only guess at what in skin causes it. Part of this youthful characteristic is likely to be due to the capillary circulation imparting a pinkish background to the skin. Another factor accounting for the distinctive appearance is the way that light reflects off and is diffused by the stratum corneum. Clearly the optical properties of this structure will change in old age as a consequence of its decreased water content and slightly increased surface roughness.

Alterations to epidermal dendritic cells

Pigment-producing melanocytes in the basal layer of the epidermis show a gradual reduction in numbers in non-exposed skin with increasing years. Studies of the numbers of Dopa-positive cells in separated epidermal whole-mount preparations suggest that there is a linear reduction of 10–20 per cent per decade.[21-23] Not only are there fewer melanocytes per unit length of epidermis, but those cells that do remain also seem smaller with a less-extensive system of dendrites. In addition to these signs of attrition of structure in the pigmentary system, the melanocytes appear less able to produce melanin pigmentation after stimulation by UVR.

Langerhans' cell numbers are also reduced in non-exposed areas of skin with increasing years. As with melanocytes the Langerhan's cells are also reduced in size and the dendrite extensions to the cells are likewise considerably reduced. There were some 15 per cent fewer Langerhans' cells in the buttock skin of subjects aged 65 or greater compared with the numbers found in a central group aged 24 or less.[24] It is not known to what extent this change in Langerhans' cell prominence accounts for the reduction in delayed hypersensitivity reactions in the elderly, as many elements of both the afferent and the efferent limbs are affected by the aging process (see later).

Age changes in the dermis

The connective tissue elements

The whole dermis loses bulk and becomes thinner with the passing of the years. Data documenting this have only been available since multiple observations in skin thickness could be taken non-invasively using either a radiological method or by employing pulsed ultrasound in either the A-scan or B-scan modes (Figure 5.8).[25-27] This gradual reduction in dermal thickness is best appreciated in non-sun-exposed sites, as in some severely sun-damaged areas there is a tendency for the skin to thicken (see Chapter 2). The reduction

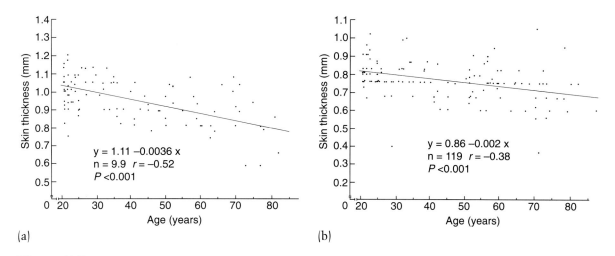

Figure 5.8

Decrease in skin thickness in (a) men and (b) women over the age of 21. (Tan CY, Stratham B, Marks R et al, Skin thickness measurement by pulsed ultrasound: Its reproducibility, validation and variability. *Br J Dermatol* (1982) **106**: 657–67).

in dermal thickness may be mainly due to reduction in the proteoglycan ground substance and as a consequence diminished water content, although all elements of dermal connective tissue are affected by the aging process.

It has been suggested that the concentration of uronic acid in sun-exposed areas of skin increases with increasing age, whereas in sun-protected skin there is a decrease of uronic acid.[28] A more recent study demonstrated a different expression of molecules of the large chondroitin sulphate proteoglycan, versican, and of the smaller proteoglycan, decorin, in photoaged and sun-protected skin.[29] Morphological analysis demonstrated a massive accumulation of versican localized to the abnormally large fibres comprising solar elastosis in the superficial dermis of actinically damaged skin. Conversely, decorin staining was greatly decreased in these areas. These findings correlated with a significant increase in versican mRNA and with fibroblast cultures derived from photodamaged skin. These results suggest that abnormal expression of the versican and decorin genes plays a role in the pathogenesis of dermal photodamage.

There is also a reduction in number and size of fibroblasts during aging as well as a decrease in their replicative attributes.[30] In addition, the collagen undergoes profound biochemical changes. There is a marked reduction in the amount of collagen per unit surface area as measured by hydroxyproline content[25] and there is a marked increase in the number of stable intermolecular cross-links with increasing age. In addition, the proportion of insoluble collagen increases while that of soluble collagen decreases.[31] The rate of collagen gene expression is reduced with advancing age.[32] The collagen is much more extensively cross-linked and thus less soluble and 'tougher', but less resilient and less extensible (see later).[33] Ultrastructural examination also reveals age related changes in the elastic fibre network. The regular fine meshwork of elastic fibres becomes less in evidence and tangles of broad and irregular fibres are seen. In addition, they tend to be more irregularly distributed in old age, more easily disrupted by enzymes, looser in texture and ragged at the edges.[34,35]

The vasculature and neural elements of the dermis share in the process of the structural attrition due to aging. The papillary capillaries decrease in numbers per unit area of skin in non-exposed sites in elderly skin. The capillary walls and basement membranes also become thinner. Laser Doppler measurement of blood flow to skin confirms what may be expected in that there is a marked decrease in the volume flow to the most superficial parts of skin with increasing age.

There is also a reduction in the number of nerve fibres and nerve endings in non-sun-exposed elderly skin, but there seem to have been few studies examining the skin's neural network and there are very few quantitative data that can illuminate this aspect of the biology of aging skin. Certainly, sensory function, for example two-point discrimination, decreases with age.

The mechanical responses of elderly skin

Some of the difficulties of characterizing the mechanical properties of skin have been pointed out previously (Chapter 2). Apart from the obvious problem of sorting out what is due to aging and what is the result of photodamage, even in well-protected sites an almost insuperable difficulty lies in determining which part of the response obtained is due to the dermal connective tissue and which is due to other tissues of and beneath the skin. Inspection of the dermis will also reveal a further confounding factor in that the dermis is itself by no means a homogeneous structure. It has clear differences in the diameters of its fibrous components and its spatial arrangements at different depths within skin. Even worse, there is often uncertainty in the mind of the investigator as to what information is actually needed. It is not often that the actual intrinsic mechanical property of a particular part of skin is the true focus of study. This parameter may be determined in vitro and the data obtained are somewhat remote from any clinical effects that changes in the figures obtained may imply. For the most part it is overall response or function of the part to mechanical stress that is of major clinical interest and importance. This overall response will be compounded by the individual mechanical properties of the epidermis and stratum corneum, the different parts of the fibrous dermal connective tissue, the non-fibrous dermal elements and the subcutaneous tissue. All the testing techniques and devices employed to examine the mechanical responsiveness of elderly skin indicate that it is markedly different mechanically from youthful skin. Suction devices including the recently introduced Cutometer[36] have been particularly helpful in delineating the differences. This interesting instrument sucks a 'bubble' of skin through a port of variable size and measures the height reached by the tip of the bubble of skin. For the most part the alterations recorded demonstrate that the extensibility of skin decreases as a function of age, i.e. it becomes stiffer and its breaking strain decreases.

The thinned dermis seems much less protective than the fuller, more resilient skin of youth and early adult life. This may be some part of the reason why tripping and falling in the elderly can be so devastating: without the full protective and cushioning effect of skin, serious injury to deeper tissues is more likely to occur. It may also contribute to the altered appearance of elderly skin, although in many instances these changes are subtle and are nowhere near as dramatic as those that occur in photodamaged skin—as well as being different in kind.

The dermo-epidermal junction

This is a complex area between the epidermis and the dermis which has an important

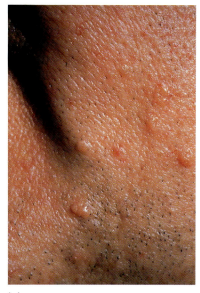

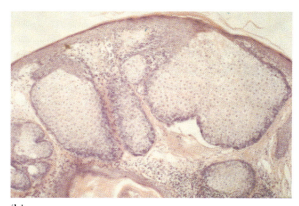

Figure 5.9

(a) Sebaceous hyperplasia on cheek of elderly man. (b) Photomicrograph of sebaceous gland hyperplasia in biopsy of lesion from forehead (H. and E. ×45).

controlling influence on skin biology and is the target of a number of disease processes. Detailed ultrastructural studies indicate that at least below the age of 60 the width of the basal lamina is unrelated to chronological age, although there seems to be an age-dependent decrease in the number of dermal microfibril bundles.[37]

Sebaceous and sweat glands

Sebaceous glands do not seem to decrease in size in the elderly. Indeed there seems to be a paradoxical increase in size of these fascinating adnexal structures in some individuals in old age. In men, on the head and neck and upper trunk in particular, the sebaceous glands tend to enlarge. Clinically the hypertrophic glands are clinically evident as small (2–4 mm diameter) orange-yellow nodules that are often mistaken for basal cell carcinoma (Figure 5.9). There is no adequate explanation for this phenomenon and it seems unlikely that solar exposure is the complete or even a partial explanation. The rate of sebum secretion does not decrease until the age of 80 or thereabouts in men, but seems to decrease in women after the menopause.[38] Both eccrine and apocrine glands decrease in size in old age. They may accumulate granules of lipofuscin in the glandular epithelium—the significance of which is unknown. The rates of sweat secretion in response to stimuli is decreased in the elderly.

Inflammation and wound healing in aged skin

One tends to think of skin of the elderly citizen as being vulnerable and easily inflamed. The situation is, in fact, somewhat more complicated. As pointed out earlier, elderly skin is more readily injured mechanically and because of the diminished immune defences is more vulnerable to microbial invasion. Curiously, though, the skin of the elderly responds to such insults with somewhat less inflammation than would be elicited from a younger individual in receipt of the same degree of trauma. As pointed out by Cook and Dzubow in a comprehensive review of the effects of aging on the healing of cutaneous wounds, incision lines are less red, the scarring is less hypertrophic and 'normalisation of appearance occurs more rapidly'.[39] In addition, the threshold at which an inflammatory response occurs is significantly higher in the older subject. Thus, the threshold to the development of erythema after irradiation with UVR is increased[40] and the reaction after treating the skin with sodium lauryl sulphate is diminished compared with that in the young.[41] Similarly, raising blisters on the skin of the elderly with suction[42] takes longer and is more difficult. In fact to quote Kligman and Bolin 'without belabouring the tissue, it can be stated categorically that acute inflammatory reactions of all kinds are muted and reduced in the aged'.[43]

The reasons for this type of diminished reactivity to trauma are uncharacterized, but are likely to be at least in part the compound result of decreased vascularity and a decreased ability to vasodilate those vessels which remain functional. In addition, cell mobility is reduced in the elderly, so that inflammatory cells accumulate less extensively and somewhat more slowly, as well as producing cytokines and mediators less efficiently.

Whatever the reasons for the lessened inflammatory response to a stimulus, the combination of increased vulnerability to various traumas and the reduced inflammatory responses is potentially dangerous and explains why skin infections such as erysipelas in the elderly can spread with such alarming rapidity and may result in death.

Immune responses are also decreased in elderly subjects and once again this seems multifactorial in origin. The number of 'patch test positives' appears to decrease with age[44] and it is certainly more difficult to sensitize elderly subjects with potent antigens such as dinitrochlorobenzene (DNCB).[45] Certainly, allergic contact dermatitis seems less of a clinical problem in the elderly than in young and mature adults. Of course, the older age group is less frequently exposed to chemical assault in the 'workplace' and this may in part also account for the decreased problem. Furthermore, and as already pointed out, the numbers of Langerhans' cells in the epidermis decrease with age. Lymphocyte activities are also compromised in the elderly.[46] It appears that both the afferent and the efferent limbs of the delayed hypersensitivity cellular immune response are defective in old age. The detail of the depressed delayed hypersensitivity is far from complete, although the broad general outlines are well documented. The same cannot be said for immediate hypersensitivity, where there seems to be very little in the way of validated data as to what happens to this component of the immune system in the aging process. All that can be said is that in general the frequency and vigour of immediate hypersensitivity reactions appear decreased.[47,48] Interestingly, the level and speed of antibody response after immunization does not appear to be compromised in old age.

Wound healing is a complex but primitive response to all kinds of trauma, mechanical and toxic. After the initial haemostasis cell migration, mitotic activity and remodelling occur in an elegant series of tissue interactions.

It has often been suggested that wounds take longer to heal in the elderly—perhaps partially explaining the fact of surgical wounds taking longer to heal and the sluggish healing of leg ulcers in this age group. While this may be the case, there have not been a great many reports to support this observation. An intriguing and detailed report was that of a military surgeon in the First World War who observed that wounds healed more rapidly in younger soliders than in those more advanced in years.[49]

More recently it has been reported that experimental wounds take longer to re-epithelialize with increasing age of the subject. Blister bases took longer to re-epithelialize in elderly

Intrinsic aging of skin

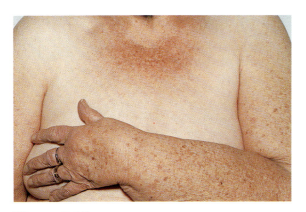

Figure 5.10
Photodamaged forearm across upper chest.

human subjects than in younger age groups.[50] Taking what has been said above concerning the altered biology of senescent skin and the depressed inflammatory responses of the elderly, it would perhaps be surprising if wound healing too was not somewhat reduced in vigour and speed in the elderly. The repair and remodelling of dermal connective tissue may also result in weaker scars in the elderly compared with younger individuals.

Intrinsic aging and photoaging contrasted

It is quite difficult to distinguish solar damage from intrinsic aging because the deleterious

Table 5.1 Intrinsic aging and photoaging contrasted

Feature	*Intrinsically aged (covered skin)*	*Chronically photodamaged (exposed skin)*
Clinical	Pale, smooth, looks and feels thin. Sparse, thin, grey hair and thin, brittle nails.	Irregularly pigmented, coarse and wrinkled. May have background of sallow, yellowish, leathery appearance. Studded with solar keratoses, senile lentigines, purpuric spots and triradiate scars.
Epidermis	Epidermis becomes thinner and flatter in profile with increasing age. Keratinocytes become smaller. Corneocytes develop larger surface area. Stratum corneum unchanged in thickness. Rate of cell production slightly decreased or unchanged. Melanocytes and Langerhans' cells decreased in number, size and activity.	Epidermis thickens irregularly, finally after extreme photodamage becomes atrophic and thinner. Focal irregularities and changes of dysplasia occur. Proliferative rate is increased. No stratum corneum change. Melanocytes and melanin production increased irregularly. Langerhans' cells decrease in number, size and activity.
Dermis	Dermis thins with increasing age. Collagen becomes more insoluble and develops more cross-links. Becomes stiffer and less extensible. Decrease in fibroblast numbers.	Dermis may become irregularly thickened due to deposition of proteoglycan. Elastotic material deposited in upper and mid-dermis. Mechanical properties markedly change.
Inflammatory response and wound healing	Diminished inflammatory responses to all types of trauma. Diminished rate of wound healing.	Diminished vasculature. Diminished inflammatory cell function.

effects of chronic actinic irradiation are superimposed on the effects of the intrinsic aging process. However, the visible alterations due to UVR damage are more dramatic and extensive in most sun-exposed sites, and swamp the more subtle changes due to intrinsic aging. Clinically the differences are easily seen if the photodamaged forearm is photographed against the sun-protected upper chest (Figure 5.10). The habitually exposed areas of the face, neck and dorsum of hands appear wrinkled, mottled, thickened and leathery. The presence of solar keratoses adds to the appearance and sensation of increased roughness and irregularity, although in fact the skin surface contour is somewhat flatter in chronically sun-damaged skin than in intrinsically aged skin (see page 87). In contrast, sun-protected skin appears evenly pale, smooth and blemish-free. Table 5.1 contrasts some of the clinical, histological and physiological features of intrinsically aged and chronically photodamaged skin.

References

1. Torras H. Retinoids in aging. In: Ledo A (ed). *Clinics in Dermatology. Skin aging and photoaging* (1996) **14**: 207–15.
2. Tanaka M, Gong JS, Zhang J et al, Mitochondrial genotype associated with longevity. *Lancet* (1998) **351**: 185–6.
3. Allsop RC, Harley CB, Evidence for a critical telomere length in senescent human fibroblasts. *Exp Cell Res* (1995) **219**: 130–6.
4. Wynn RF, Cross MA, Hatton C et al, Accelerated telomere shortening in young recipients of allogenic bone-marrow transplants. *Lancet* (1998) **351**: 178–81.
5. Hayflick L, The cell biology of human aging. *Sci Am* (1980) **242**: 58–66.
6. Darr D, Fridovich I, Free radical sin cutaneous biology. *J Invest Dermatol* (1994) **102**: 671–5.
7. Marks R, Measurement of biological aging in human epidermis. *Br J Dermatol* (1981) **104**: 627–33.
8. Plewig G, Marples RR, Regional differences of cell sizes in human stratum corneum Part II. Effects of aging and sex. *J Invest Dermatol* (1970) **54**: 19–23.
9. Grove G, Lavker RM, Holzle E, Kligman AM, Use of non intrusive tests to monitor age associated changes in human skin. *J Soc Cos Chem* (1981) **32**: 15–19.
10. Wilhelm KP, Cua AB, Maibach HI, Effect of age on transepidermal water loss, stratum corneum hydration, skin surface pH and casual sebum content. *Arch Dermatol* (1991) **127**: 1806–9.
11. Marks R, Barton SP, The significance of the size and shape of corneocytes. In: R Marks, G Plewig (eds) *Stratum Corneum.* Springer-Verlag: Berlin, 1983, pp. 153–60.
12. Roberts D, Marks R, Determination of regional and age variations in the rate of desquamation. Comparison of four techniques. *J Invest Dermatol* (1979) **74**: 13–16.
13. Kligman AM, Perspectives and problems in cutaneous gerontology. *J Invest Dermatol* (1979) **73**: 39–46.
14. Edwards CE, Heggie RH, Marks R, A study of differences in surface roughness between exposed and unexposed skin with age. (In press.)
15. Lavker RM, Kwang F, Kligman AM, Changes in skin surface pattern with age. *J Gerontol* (1980) **35**: 348–54.
16. Potts RO, Buras EM, Chrisman DA, Changes with age in the moisture content of human skin. *J Invest Dermatol* (1984) **82**: 97–100.
17. Silver AF, Montagna AW, Karacan I, The effect of age on human eccrine sweating. In: W Montagna (ed.) *Advances in Biology of the Skin*, Vol IV. Pergamon Press: Oxford, 1965, pp. 129–50.
18. Pochi PE, Strauss JS, Dowing DT, Age related changes in sebaceous gland activity. *J Invest Dermatol* (1979) **73**: 108–111.
19. Giacometti L, Hair growth and aging. In: W Montagna (ed.) *Advances in Biology of the Skin*, Vol VI. Pergamon Press: Oxford, 1965, pp. 97–118.
20. Bean WB, Nail growth. Twenty five years observation. *Arch Int Med* (1968) **122**: 359–61.
21. Fitzpatrick TB, Szabo G, Mitchell RE, Age changes in the human melanocyte system. In:

W Montagna (ed.) *Advances in Biology of the Skin*. Pergamon Press: Oxford, 1964.
22. Quevedo WC, Szabo G, Virks J, Influence of age and UV on the population of dopa-positive melanocytes in human skin. *J Invest Dermatol* (1969) **52**: 287–90.
23. Snell RS, Bischitz PG, The melanocytes and melanin in human abdominal wall skin. A survey made at different ages in both sexes and in pregnancy. *J Anat* (1979) **97**: 361–76.
24. Thiers BH, Maize JC, Spicer S et al, The effect of aging and chronic sun exposure on human Langerhans cell population. *J Invest Dermatol* (1984) **82**: 223–6.
25. Shuster S, Black MM, McVitie E, The influence of age and sex on skin thickness, skin collagen and density. *Br J Dermatol* (1975) **93**: 639–43.
26. Tan CY, Stratham B, Marks R et al, Skin thickness measurement by pulsed ultrasound: Its reproducibility, validation and variability. *Br J Dermatol* (1982) **106**: 657–67.
27. De Rigal J, Escoffier C, Querleux B et al, Assessment of skin aging of human skin by in vivo ultrasonic imaging. *J Invest Dermatol* (1989) **93**: 621–5.
28. Johnston KJ, Oikarinen AI, Lowe NJ, Uitto J, Ultraviolet induced connective tissue changes in the skin: Models for actinic damage and cutaneous aging. In: HI Maibach, NJ Lowe (eds) *Models in Dermatology*, Vol I. Karger: Basel, 1985, pp. 69–76.
29. Bernstein EF, Fisher LW, Lik et al, Differential expression of the versican and decorin genes in photoaged and sun protected skin. *Lab Invest* (1995) **72**: 662–9.
30. Schneider EL, Aging and cultured human skin fibroblasts. *J Invest Dermatol* (1979) **73**: 15–18.
31. Hall DA, *The Aging of Connective Tissue*. Academic Press: London, 1976.
32. Uitto J, Fazio MJ, Olsen DR, Molecular mechanisms of cutaneous aging. *J Am Acad Dermatol* (1989) **21**: 614–22.
33. Escoffier CE, de Rigal J, Rochefort A et al, Age related mechanical properties of human skin: An in vivo study. *J Invest Dermatol* (1989) **93**: 353–7.
34. Braverman IM, Forfeko E, Studies in cutaneous aging: I: the elastic fiber network. *J Invest Dermatol* (1982) **78**: 434–43.
35. Tsiyi T, Hamada T, Age related changes in human dermal elastic fibres. *Br J Dermatol* (1981) **105**: 57–63.
36. Pierard GE, Kort R, Letawe C et al, Biomechanical assessment of photodamage. Derivation of a cutaneous extrinsic aging score. *Skin Res and Tech* (1995) **1**: 17–20.
37. Tidman MJ, Eady RAJ, Ultrastructural morphometry of normal human dermal-epidermal junction. The influence of age, sex and body region on laminar and non laminar components. *J Invest Dermatol* (1984) **83**: 448–53.
38. Pochi PE, Strauss JS, Downing DT, Age related changes in sebaceous gland activity. *J Invest Dermatol* (1979) **73**: 108–11.
39. Cook JL, Dzubow LM, Aging of the skin. Implications for cutaneous surgery. *Arch Dermatol* (1997) **133**: 1273–7.
40. Gilchrest BA, Stoff JS, Soter NA, Chronologic aging alters the response to UV induced inflammation in human skin. *J Invest Dermatol* (1982) **79**: 11–16.
41. Grove GL, Lavker RM, Holzel E, Kligman AM, Use of non intrusive tests to monitor age associated changes in human skin. *J Soc Cos Chem* (1981) **32**: 15–26.
42. Kiistala U, Dermoepidermal separation. The effects of age, sex and body region on suction blister formation. *Ann Clin Res* (1972) **4**: 10–22.
43. Kligman AM, Balin AK, Aging of human skin. In: AM Kligman, AK Bolin (eds) *Aging and the Skin*. Raven Press: New York, 1988, pp. 1–42.
44. Leyman E, Stoudemayer T, Grove G et al, Age differences in poison ivy dermatitis. *Cont Derm* (1984) **11**: 163–7.
45. Catalona WJ, Taylor PT, Rabson AS, Chretein PB, A method of dinitrochlorobenzene sensitization: A clinicopathological study. *N Engl J Med* (1972) **286**: 399–406.
46. Hallgren HM, Kersey JH, Dubey DP, Yunis EJ, Lymphocyte subsets and integrated immune function in aging human. *Clin Immunol Immunopathol* (1978) **10**: 65–78.
47. Marsh DG, Meyer DA, The epidemiology of atopic allergy. *N Engl J Med* (1981) **305**: 1551–60.
48. Sunderkotter C, Kalden H, Luger TA, Aging and the skin immune system. *Arch Dermatol* (1997) **133**: 1256–62.

49. DuNouy PL, *Biological Time*. MacMillan: New York, 1937.

50. Grove GL, Age related differences in healing of superficial skin wounds in humans. *Arch Derm Res* (1982) **272**: 381–85.

6 The effects of sun exposure on the immune response

Introduction

Conventional wisdom suggests that spending time in the sun enhances fitness and resistance to disease. This view appears to be supported by the antimicrobial action of ultraviolet (UVC), which is exploited in sterilizing cabinets, and in the use of the disinfecting properties of sunlight on water for the purification of drinking water.[1] There are certainly some psychological benefits and maybe transient therapeutic benefits too for some skin disorders such as acne[2] and psoriasis.[3] Sun exposure is also vital to the synthesis of vitamin D_3 via the action of solar ultraviolet irradiation (UVR) on cholecalciferol in the epidermis. Vitamin D_3 is required for bone metabolism and growth and without it rickets or osteomalacia develops. Vitamin D_3 also appears important in the resistance to microbial disease, and the generation of this compound by UVR may have been the mechanism of action of the 'Finsen light' treatment for cutaneous tuberculosis and the solarium and heliotherapy treatments for pulmonary tuberculosis. In fact comparatively little sun exposure is needed to prevent rickets or osteomalacia—of the order of 30 minutes on a summer's day twice weekly in a temperate climate in ordinary Western-style clothes.[4]

Unfortunately most of the rest of the evidence as to the effects of sun exposure on the immune system seems to point in a negative direction and forms the basis of the recently developed science of photoimmunology and the substance of this chapter.

At the outset it should be pointed out that the subject is developing rapidly and that new information may rapidly supersede the information given below. It is also the case that apart from the involvement of solar UVR in the photodermatoses and lupus erythematosis (LE), the clinical relevance of some of the immunological changes described in experimental animals or that occur in sun-exposed skin is quite unclear. One reason for this may be that the immunosuppression caused by exposure to solar UVR predisposes to disease, but it is not itself visible.[5] It is difficult to know to what degree the immunosuppression caused will contribute to disease. How much, for example, does immunosuppression contribute to the development of a squamous cell carcinoma compared with the direct changes in nuclear DNA caused by exposure to solar UVR?

Most of the data generated on the effects of UV energy on the immune system come from studies on small mammals. As most of these experimental animals are furry and their skin

Effects of UVR on delayed hypersensitivity

The earliest observations were made on guinea-pigs[6] and mice,[7] in which it was observed that irradiation by artificial sources of UVR caused tolerance of antigens if the application of the antigens were made to previously UV-irradiated skin. Furthermore, specific tolerance to the potent allergen in question could be induced in naive animals by transfer of T lymphocytes from the UVR-induced anergic animal. These results were obtained with low-intensity UV radiation—an important issue, as with a high UVR flux somewhat different results were obtained. When mice were given high-intensity UVR, anergy to a particular hapten was found on both irradiated and non-irradiated sites.[8] In addition, immunosuppression to other antigens was detected, both phenomena suggesting a systemic influence from the UV radiation.[9]

The variation in the severity of photodamage in different individuals is only partially explained by the depth of their skin pigmentation. This applies to all the different UVR-induced effects on the skin and almost certainly applies to UVR-induced immunosuppression as well. For this reason the study reported by Noonan and Hoffman[10] was of special interest, as they reported that mice differed considerably in their susceptibility to UVR-induced immunosuppression and that this immunosuppression appeared to be under the genetic control of interacting autosomal dominant and X-linked genes. Whether or not delayed hypersensitivity will develop when an allergen is applied to UV-treated skin of mice also seems to depend on other genetic factors, including polymorphism of the tumour necrosis factor-α gene.[11]

UVR exposure: the immune response and photocarcinogenesis

The anergy induced by UVR in experimental animals may be of great importance in photocarcinogenesis. In a classic series of experiments by Kripke and her colleagues it was shown that when neoplastic lesions induced in mice by UVR were transplanted into genetically identical animals their growth was facilitated by injecting the mice with spleen cells from the UVR-irradiated mice.[8] Furthermore, when mice are chronically exposed to UVR they lose their ability to mount an immunological response to UV-induced neoplasms.[12] Such a result indicates that the irradiation induced a specific acquired lymphocyte-mediated anergy. Clearly this has important implications for the development of non-melanoma skin cancer in light-exposed areas in man and possibly for distant non-light-exposed sites as well. With regard to this latter issue, it was worrying to read the report of Bentham (1988),[13] which concluded that the incidence of non-Hodgkin's lymphoma in different areas of the UK was positively associated with levels of ambient UVR. This author suggests that the results of this study were consistent with the hypothesis that exposure to solar UVR 'increased the risk of non-Hodgkin's lymphoma'. Other authors have shared Bentham's view,[14,15] but at least one American group do not subscribe to this suggestion. Freedman et al[16] could not identify an association of non-Hodgkin's lymphoma with increased exposure to solar UVR in the USA, despite confirming the association with skin cancer.

The drug-induced immunosuppression in patients who have had renal transplants is generally acceded to be the major reason for greatly increased numbers of non-melanoma skin cancers (NMSCs) in this group.[17-19] As persistent UVR exposure directly causes damage to and mutations in DNA (see Chapter 4) and at the same time suppresses delayed hypersensitivity, it seem likely that this double mechanism may account for the many skin cancers seen in badly sun-damaged individuals.

An important and early observation which is surely highly relevant to the effects of UVR on delayed hypersensitivity was the observed effect of UVB on Langerhans' cells. Several studies have reported that after exposure to UVB Langerhans' cells in the skin show a decreased in numbers[20,21] as assessed by several of the various Langerhans' cell-labelling techniques available. Sunburning doses of UVB (greater than 1000 J/m^2) cause Langerhans' cells to lose their dendritic processes. The Langerhans' cells also lose some of their surface markers, including MHC class II complexes as well as ATPase activity, in both mouse and human skin. The clear implication of all this is that defective Langerhans' cell function from UVR exposure will mean that when an antigen is applied to the skin it will not be presented to T cells and will result in failure to mount a delayed hypersensitivity response to it.

Interestingly enough, irradiation with UVB has been shown to inhibit the ability of Langerhans' cells to stimulate one subpopulation of lymphocytes—TH1 cells—but has no effect on their ability to activate TH2 cells, another lymphocyte subpopulation. As the latter secrete IL-4, IL-5 and IL-10 and are responsible for facilitating B cell function, while the former predominantly secrete IL-2 and interferon γ and are mainly concerned with delayed hypersensitivity, it can be seen that UVB irradiation that does not completely kill all Langerhans' cells will substantially alter the pattern of the immune response.

There can be little doubt that Langerhans' cell function is altered after exposure to UVR. There has, however, been some dispute as to whether these marrow-deprived dendritic cells are actually decreased in number or not after irradiation. The difficulty has been the multiplicity of animal species studied, the different UVR dosage regimens used and the various methods employed to quantify the numbers of Langerhans' cells. A fascinating study by Van Praag et al[22] in which human volunteers were irradiated over a 4-week period did not detect a reduction in Langerhans' cell numbers using an immuno-electron microscopic technique, even though there was a pronounced reduction in the mixed epidermal cell lymphocyte reaction indicating a diminished delayed hypersensitivity response.

It has been suggested that TH-2-derived IL-10 may be responsible for the continuing suppression of TH-1 cells.[11] Antibodies to IL-10 have been shown to inhibit the UVB-induced reduced delayed hypersensitivity response in mice. In addition, mice which lack expression of IL-10 (IL-10 gene-targeted) were found to be resistant to UVB-induced immunosuppression, although not resistant to immunosuppression of contact hypersensitivity at a site distant from that irradiated.[23] Clearly IL-10 plays an extremely important role in UVB-induced immunosuppression.

It seems that CD11b-positive monocyte macrophages also play a role in UVR-induced immune tolerance, as the findings in one study indicated that a monoclonal antibody directed against these cells restored the contact hypersensitivity response[24] after UVR-induced immunosuppression.

In another study the role of another interleukin was investigated. Administration of IL-12 intraperitoneally was found to prevent UVR-induced immunosuppression in mice sensitized to dinitrofluorobenzene.[25] Presumably this is due to the involvement of IL-12 in the development of TH-1 cells that are vital to delayed hypersensitivity. Perhaps not surprisingly, the vasodilatory mediators nitric oxide (NO) and calcitonin gene-related peptide (CGRP) are both released in the skin after UVR and it has recently been demonstrated that these mediators are also involved in the immunosuppression due to UVR by use of specific inhibitors of the NO and CGRP synthesis.[26]

Other UV effects on the immune response

UVR seems to have a curious effect on the distribution of lymphocytes. In UV-irradiated small mammals there appears to be a redistribution of lymphocytes in that there are increased numbers in the lymph nodes, but the functional significance of this is uncertain.

A further potential immunomodulating effect of UVR is the influence that UVR has on the relative proportions of the *cis*- and *trans*-isomers of urocanic acid. Urocanic acid is one of the compounds generated from filaggrin in the upper epidermis during differentiation. UVR stimulates the conversion of the *trans*-isomer of urocanic acid to the *cis*-form and this latter compound has immunosuppressive properties. There is evidence that this process of photoisomerization resulting in increased amounts of the *cis*-isomer of urocanic acid suppresses delayed hypersensitivity in mice.[27] *Cis*-urocanic acid seems to inhibit the antigen-presenting function of spleen dendritic cells.[28] Deletion of the in vivo action of *cis*-urocanic acid by injection of a monoclonal antibody against this isomer prevented the suppression of delayed hypersensitivity reactions, but had no effect on the suppression of contact hypersensitivity.[29] The kinetics of IL-10 expression in the skin was also altered by the anti-*cis*-urocanic acid antibody. It appears that this action of UVR on the proportions of the *cis*- and *trans*-isomers of urocanic acid affects only part of the immunosuppressive mechanism, but the place of this fascinating UVR-driven immunosuppression in the overall immunological profile after UVR exposure in man is unclear. As pointed out, the clinical relevance of many of the studies reported in this relatively new area of photoimmunology is unknown, but one study in which a clear message for human biology is given should be quoted. In this study by Cestari and colleagues from Brazil, lepromin-positive healthy contacts of leprosy patients were tested with lepromin in both UV-irradiated (2 minimal erythema doses (MED) every 4 days over 3 weeks) or control sites. The lepromin-induced granulomas were significantly smaller with lesser numbers of CD4-positive T cells in the lesions in irradiated skin.[30]

Photodermatoses and photoimmunological effects

There are a number of skin disorders which are the result of exposure to solar UVR and in which the immune system is intimately involved in the pathogenesis. The detail of the immunopathogenesis in most cases is not fully elucidated and only brief comments on the mechanisms involved will be made here. These disorders include Hutchinson's summer prurigo (actinic prurigo), polymorphic light eruption, solar urticaria, chronic actinic dermatitis and the drug photosensitivities.

Hutchinson's summer prurigo

This curious disorder is an itchy, eczematous eruption (Figure 6.1) appearing in the light-exposed areas of young females usually below the age of 15 and remitting before the age of

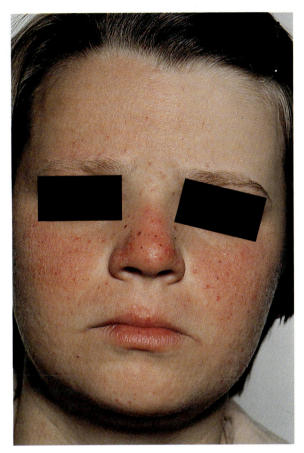

Figure 6.1
Actinic prurigo in 13 year old.

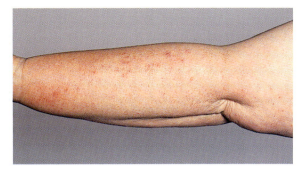

Figure 6.2
Polymorphic light eruption in middle-aged woman.

30. It does have strong clinical resemblance to atopic dermatitis with excortication and lichenification as well as scaling and papules. It has a hereditary basis in some patients with evidence that the haplotype HLA-DR4 confers genetic susceptibility to the disease in Caucasians. There is also a strong inherited susceptibility in some American Indian groups, where other major histocompatibility antigens appear to be involved.[31] Light testing does not usually implicate a specific wavelength and treatment is directed to sun avoidance and symptom control.

Polymorphic light eruption (PLE)

This disorder is much more common than is generally thought. Some authors suggesting that as much as 10 or even 15 per cent of the population are affected at some time to some degree.[32,33] PLE, as its name suggests, has different clinical manifestations in different patients. Papules, papulovesicles, nodules and plaques may all be seen (Figure 6.2). It mostly develops first in young adult life but can have a late onset in a few patients. The disorder usually develops on exposed skin after 2 or 3 days of sunny weather and tends to improve later in the summer.

PLE is thought of as a delayed hypersensitivity reaction to a solar-induced antigen. In favour of this concept are its delayed onset and the histological appearance of a perivascular lymphocyte infiltrate, as well as spongiosis and a pattern of adhesion molecule expression as seen in cutaneous delayed hypersensitivity reactions.[34]

Patients with PLE often react to wavelengths in the UVA range, but this is not invariable and some react to UVB wavelengths. Treatment is by avoidance of UV exposure and use of UVA sunscreens. Some patients, but not all, are helped by β-carotene and antimalarials. Topical corticosteroids provide some temporary relief.

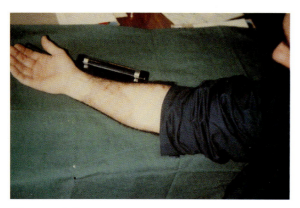

Figure 6.3
Solar urticaria. An urticarial area has been induced on the forearm of this patient with solar urticaria with a portable black light UVR lamp.

'Hardening' by repeated sun exposure or a course of PUVA before the summer season begins is also of help.

Solar urticaria

This disorder is quite uncommon and is evoked by exposure to specific wavelengths in the UVA, UVB or visible light wavebands. Urticarial lesions develop on exposed sites within a minute or two and last for up to 2 hours after exposure (Figure 6.3). It has been suggested that the disorder is a form of immediate hypersensitivity to a sun-induced photoallergen.

Patients should avoid the sun, use appropriate sunscreens and take H_1-blocking antihistamines. If these measures do not help, gradually increasing exposure to the evocative wavelength(s) every year markedly diminishes the reactions they produce and makes life at least tolerable.

Care should be taken to differentiate this disorder form erythropoietic protoporphysia in which urticaria-like lesions may occur by protoporphyrin estimations.

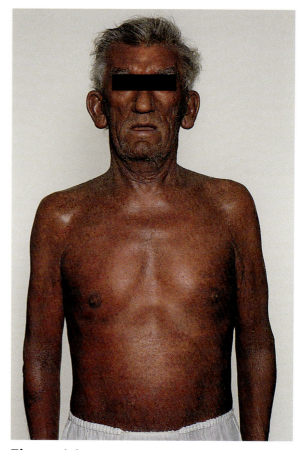

Figure 6.4
Chronic actinic dermatitis of 18 months duration. He was exquisitely sensitive to light exposure.

Chronic actinic dermatitis (CAD)

Chronic actinic dermatitis (CAD) has in the past been called 'photosensitive eczema', 'persistent light reaction' and 'actinic reticuloid', but by consensus is now only referred to as CAD. It is an odd disease which predominantly affects middle-aged or elderly men, causing eczematous, lichenified and plaque-like lesions to develop mainly on exposed areas (Figure 6.4), although in some patients much more widespread lesions develop. In some patients the thickening of the skin and

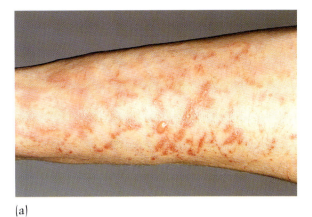 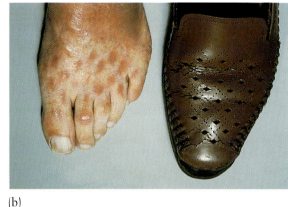

(a) (b)

Figure 6.5

(a) Phytophotodermatitis of arm after coming into contact with plant juice while gardening. (b) Photosensitivity in man with chronic actinic dermatitis. The reaction has occurred beneath the holes in his shoe.

the dense and 'activated' cellular infiltrate has some similarities to a cutaneous reticulosis, which is how the name 'actinic reticuloid' developed.

The disease was first noticed after the epidemic of photosensitivity eczema caused by the halogenated salicylanilides (particularly tetrachlorsalicylanilide [TCSA]) in soaps. It is thought that CAD is initiated by photocontact sensitization to a compound such as TCSA and subsequently is 'self-generating' in that no further contact with the compound to which photosensitivity developed is necessary—just light. Although the initiating photosensitizing wavelength is usually in the UVA range, progression to 'mature CAD' is marked by a change in photosensitivity to the UVB waveband and longer wavelengths. Other photobiological features include exquisite light sensitivity with a marked reduction in minimal erythema dose and reaction to some visible light wavelengths.

Many patients have positive photocontact reactions to composite oleoresins and fragrance materials.[35] A study of the appearance of adhesion molecules in induced lesions shows these to be similar to those found in type IV hypersensitivity.[36]

Management of this disorder can be very difficult as many patients are so supersensitive that they must be nursed in semi-darkness. Topical agents including corticosteroids are not generally of much help and most require systemic steroids, azathioprine or cyclosporin.

Photosensitivity and phototoxicity to exogenous materials

There are many compounds which if ingested or contacted cause the exposed skin to react with an inflamed erythematous rash after UVR exposure (Figure 6.5). Essentially, two different types of this response are recognized: the phototoxic reaction and the photosensitivity type of response or photoallergic reaction.[37] The phototoxic reaction can occur in anyone suitably exposed and responsible compounds include the psoralens, the porphyrins, coal tar, nonsteroidal anti-inflammatory drugs and antibiotics. Confusingly, some of the drugs causing phototoxicity can also elicit a photoallergic reaction. Another difficulty is the morphological similarity between the two types of response both clinically and histologically. Photoallergic responses have all the characteristics of type IV reactions and occur only in previously sensitized individuals. Examples of materials that cause a photoallergic reaction include halogenated salicylanilides, para-aminobenzoic acid derivatives, oxybenzone, musk ambrette and parsol 1789. The action spectrum for most of the photosensitivity and phototoxic disorders is in the UVA range.

Other disorders

The disorders briefly described above are due to the interaction of solar energy and the immune system and can with some justification be described as photoimmunological in origin. However, there are many other disorders which have not been described which, if not directly the result of photoimmunological interactions, are at least in part due to or are aggravated by photoimmunological influences. Lupus erythematosus (LE) is one such disease—many patients with the systemic variety recognize that exposure to the sun will result in worsening of their disease.[8] Similarly patients with discoid LE may develop new lesions or a flare-up of existing lesions if exposed to the sun.

Protection against immunosuppressive action of UVR

Can use of sunscreen or other sun protection manoeuvres prevent the changes described in the preceding pages in this chapter? The answer is complex as it depends both on the particular disorder and the type of protection used.

Such disorders as polymorphic light eruption and Hutchinson's summer prurigo are specifically sensitive to the long waves of UVR (UVA) and it is pointless giving patients with these conditions sunscreens which protect predominantly against medium wave (UVB) UVR. Use of sunscreens containing reflectant substances such as microionized titanium dioxide give some protection across the UV spectrum. This and similar agents can be helpful when incorporated into sunscreens, but some patients are so exquisitely sensitive to the sun that even this form of protection is inadequate. The protective capacity of sunscreens with regard to experimentally induced UV suppression is quite contentious. A study by Wolf et al[39] investigated three sunscreens, one containing a P-aminobenzoic acid ester, another containing a cinnamate and a third containing a benzophenone derivative. They determined whether these protective screens could protect against UV-induced inflammation and immunosuppression as assessed by sensitization to 2,4-dinitrofluorobenzene at both a UV-irradiated site and distant site. All three sunscreens gave some protection against UVR-induced inflammation, but were less effective in protecting against the systemic component of immunosuppression. It is quite important to note that protection against UVR-induced inflammation does not necessarily mean that there will also be protection against the immunosuppressive effects of UVR. It seems that different mechanisms may be involved. The implications for the development of skin cancer in individuals who believe that they are protected by the use of sunscreens is of major concern.

A gel containing an extract of *Aloe barbadensis* was found to prevent UVB-induced immunosuppression in mice if applied after each irradiation.[40] This did not appear to be due to any sunscreening effect, but seemed to preserve the Langerhan's cells and Thy-1$^+$ dendritic epidermal cells. Another protective effect which is difficult to explain is that produced by the use of topical *N*-acetyl cysteine applied 30 minutes before UVR in mice on the systemic immunosuppression otherwise observed.[41] This effect does not appear to be due to UVR absorption and at present there is not an adequate explanation for this phenomenon.

Antioxidants (free radical scavengers) such as α-tocopherol and its derivatives and ascorbic acid have also been found to be protective against photodamage. Studies in mice have demonstrated that the redness, oedema and skin sensitivity due to UV radiation are considerably reduced by application of pure α-tocopherol oil after radiation.[42] Furthermore, tocopherol sorbate significantly reduced the generation of free radicals in UV-irradiated skin in mice.[43] A combination of vitamins C and E provided good protection against sunburn cell formation in pig skin, and perhaps not surprisingly even better protection was obtained when the vitamin combination was used together with a sunscreen.[44]

References

1. Hawk JLM, Cutaneous pathology. In: RH Champion, JL Burton, FJG Ebling (eds) *Textbook of Dermatology*, 5th edn. Blackwell Science: Oxford, 1996, p. 850.
2. Krutmann J, Czech W, Deipgen T et al, High dose UVA 1 therapy in the treatment of patients with atopic dermatitis. *J Am Acad Dermatol* (1990) **22**: 49–53.
3. Horio T, Skin disorders that improve by exposure to sunlight. *Clinics in Derm* (1998) **16**: 59–65.
4. Diffey BL, Ultraviolet radiation and human health. *Clin Dermatol* (1998) **16**: 83–9.
5. Bergstresser PR, Immediate and delayed effects of UVR on immune responses in skin. In: Gilchrist BA (ed.) *Photodamage*. Blackwell Science: 1995.
6. Hanniszko J, Suskind RR, The effect of ultra violet irradiation on experimental cutaneous sensitisation in guinea pigs. *J Invest Dermatol* (1963) **40**: 183.
7. Toews GB, Bergstresser PR, Streilein JW, Epidermal Langerhans cell density determines whether contact hypersensitivity or unresponsiveness follows skin painting with DNFB *J Immunol* (1995) **61**: 223–47.
8. Kripke ML, Immunology and photocarcinogenesis. New light on an old problem. *J Am Acad Dermatol* (1986) **14**: 149–55.
9. Wolf P, Donawho CK, Kripke ML, Analysis of the protective effect of different sunscreens on ultraviolet radiation induced local and systemic suppression of contact hypersensitivity and inflammatory responses in mice. *J Invest Dermatol* (1993) **100**: 254–9.
10. Noonan FP, Hoffman HA, Control of UVB immunosuppression in the mouse by autosomal and sex-linked genes. *Immunogenetics* (1994) **40**: 247–56.
11. Streilein JW, Sunlight and skin associated lymphoid tissues (SALT): if UVB is the trigger and TNFα is its mediator, what is the message? *J Invest Dermatol* (1993) **100**: 475–525.
12. Kripke ML, Effects of UV radiation on tumour immunity. *J Natl Cancer* (1990) **82**: 1392–6.
13. Bentham G, Association between incidence of non Hodgkin's lymphoma and solar ultraviolet radiation in England and Wales. *BMJ* (1996) **312**: 1128–31.
14. McMichael AJ, Giles GG, Have increases in solar ultraviolet exposure contributed to the rise in incidence of non Hodgkin's Lymphoma? *Br J Cancer* (1996) **73**: 945–50.
15. Cartwright R, McNally R, Staines A, The increasing incidence of non Hodgkin's lymphoma (NHL): the possible role of sunlight. *Leuk Lymphoma* (1994) **14**: 387–94.
16. Freedman DM, Zahm SH, Dosemica M, Residential and occupational exposure to sunlight and mortality from non Hodgkin's lymphoma: composite (threefold) case control study. *BMJ* (1997) **314**: 1451–55.
17. Shuttleworth D, Marks R, Epidermal dysplasia and skeletal deformity in congenital poikiloderma (Rothman–Thompson syndrome). *Br J Dermatol* (1987) **117**: 377–84.
18. Hartevelt MM, Bouwes Bavinck JN, Kootte AMM et al, Incidence of skin cancer after renal transplantation in the Netherlands. *Transplantation* (1990) **49**: 506–9.
19. Gupta AK, Cardella CJ, Haberman HF, Cutaneous malignant neoplasms in patients

with renal transplants. *Arch Dermatol* (1986) **122**: 1288–98.
20. Rae V, Yoshikawa T, Brüns-Slot W et al, An ultraviolet B radiation protocol for complete depletion of human epidermal Langerhans cells. *J Derm Surg Oncol* (1989) **15**: 1199–202.
21. Cooper KD, Oberhelman L, Hamilton TA et al, UV exposure reduces immunisation rates and promotes tolerance to epicutaneous antigens in humans: relationship to dose, CD1a-DR+ epidermal macrophage induction and Langerhans cell depletion. *Proc Natl Acad Sci USA* (1992) **89**: 8497–501.
22. Van Praag MCG, Mulder AA, Claas FHJ et al, Long term ultraviolet B-induced impairment of Langerhans cell function: an immunoelectron microscopic study. *Clin Exp Immunol* (1994) **95**: 73–7.
23. Beissert S, Hosoi J, Kuhn R et al, Impaired immunosuppressive response to ultraviolet radiation in interleukin-10-deficient mice. *J Invest Dermatol* (1996) **107**(4): 553–7.
24. Hammerberg C, Duraiswamy N, Cooper KD, Reversal of immunosuppression inducible through ultraviolet-exposed skin by in vivo anti-CD11b treatment. *J Immunol* (1996) **157**(12): 5254–61.
25. Schwarz A, Grabbe S, Aragane Y et al, Interleukin-12 prevents ultraviolet B-induced local immunosuppression and overcomes UVB-induced tolerance. *J Invest Dermatol* (1996) **106**: 1187–91.
26. Gillardon F, Moll I, Michel S et al, Calcitonin gene related peptide and nitric oxide are involved in ultraviolet radiation-induced immunosuppression. *Eur J Pharmacol* (1995) **293**: 395–400.
27. Kurimoto I, Streilein JW, *Cis*-urocanic acid suppression of contact hypersensitivity induction is mediated via tumor necrosis factor-α. *J Immunol* (1992) **148**: 3072–78.
28. Noonan FP, DeFabo EC, Morrison H, *Cis*-urocanic acid, a product formed by ultraviolet B irradiation of the skin, initiates an antigen presentation defect in splenic dendritic cells in vivo. *J Invest Dermatol* (1988) **90**: 92–9.
29. Moodycliffe AM, Bucana CD, Kripke ML et al, Differential effects of a monoclonal antibody to *cis*-urocanic acid on the suppression of delayed and contact hypersensitivity following ultraviolet irradiation. *J Immunol* (1996) **157**: 2891–9.
30. Cestari FF, Kripke ML, Baptista PL et al, Ultraviolet radiation decreases the granulomatous response to lepromin in humans. *J Invest Dermatol* (1995) **105**: 8–13.
31. Hojyo-Tomoka T, Granados J, Granados-Alaveon G et al, Further evidence of the role of HLA-DR4 in the genetic susceptibility to actinic prurigo. *J Am Acad Dermatol* (1997) **36**: 935–7.
32. Miroson WL, Stern RS, Polymorphous light eruption: a common reaction uncommonly recognised. *Acta Derm Venereol* (1982) **62**: 237–40.
33. Foriades J, Soter NA, Lim HW, Results of evaluation of 203 patients for photosensitivity in a 7.3 year period. *J Am Acad Dermatol* (1985) **33L**: 597–602.
34. Wolf R, Oumeish OY, Photodermatoses. *Clin Dermatol* (1998) **16**: 41–57.
35. Menagé H du P, Ross JS, Norris PG et al, Contact and photocontact sensitization in chronic actinic dermatitis: sesquiterpene lactone mix is an important allergen. *Br J Dermatol* (1995) **132**: 543–7.
36. Menagé H du P, Sattar NK, Haskard DO et al, A study of the kinetics and pattern of E. selectin VCAM-1 and ICAM-1 expression in chronic actinic dermatitis. *Br J Dermatol* (1996) **134**: 262–8.
37. Gould JW, Mercurio MG, Elmets CA, Cutaneous photosensitivity diseases induced by exogenous agents. *J Am Acad Dermatol* (1995) **33**: 351–73.
38. Lim HW, Epstein J, Photosensitivity diseases. *J Am Acad Dermatol* (1997) **36**: 84–90.
39. Wolf P, Yarosh DB, Kripke ML, Effects of sunscreens and a DNA excision repair enzyme on ultraviolet radiation induced inflammation, immune suppression, and cyclobutane pyrimidine dimer formation in mice. *J Invest Dermatol* (1993) **101**: 523–7.
40. Stickland FM, Pelley RP, Kripke ML, Prevention of ultraviolet radiation-induced suppression of contact and delayed hypersensitivity by *Aloe barbadensis* gel extract. *J Invest Dermatol* (1994) **120**: 197–204.
41. van den Broeke LT, Beijersbergen van Henegouwen GM, Topically applied *N*-acetylcysteine as a protector against UVB-induced systemic immunosuppression. *J Photochem Photobiol* (1995) **27**: 61–5.

42. Trevithick JR, Xiong H, Lee S et al, Topical tocopherol acetate reduces post UVB, sunburn associated erythema, edema, and skin sensitivity in hairless mice. *Arch Biochem Biophys* (1992) **296**: 575–82.
43. Jurkiewiez BA, Bissett DL, Buettner GR, Effect of topically applied tocopherol on ultraviolet radiation mediated free radical damage in skin. *J Invest Dermatol* (1995) **104**: 484–8.
44. Darr D, Dunston S, Faust H, Pinnell S, Effectiveness of antioxidants (vitamin C and E) with an without sunscreens as topical photoprotectants. *Acta Derm Venereol* (1996) **76**: 264–8.

7 The measurement of photodamage

Introduction

Photodamage is only too evident clinically. Why measure it? Is it in fact possible to measure photodamage accurately, reproducibly and conveniently? The answer to the first question is the same as that which should be given to any similar enquiry applied to any other area of medicine. Measurement is helpful (some would say essential) to provide an objective and quantative assessment of the severity of the disease process in order to provide a permanent 'hard copy' historical record. Amongst other things, taking a measurement is also an important aid to the assessment of the efficacy of a treatment. Measurement of the extent of tissue damage also allows characterization of the relationships and correlations between photodamage, external stimuli and personal characteristics and susceptibilities. In this short chapter we will review both structural and functional changes found in photodamaged skin and describe the techniques available to measure the degree of abnormality present.

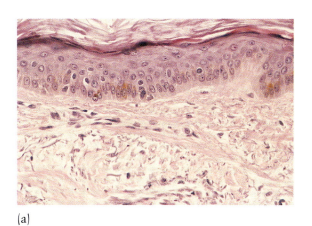
(a)

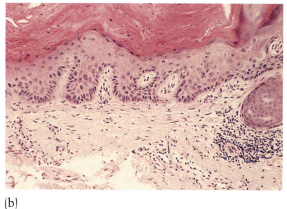
(b)

Figure 7.1

Two examples of minimal dysplasia in biopsies of sun-damaged skin. There is some heterogeneity of cell size and shape and staining and some loss of cell polarity (H. and E. ×90).

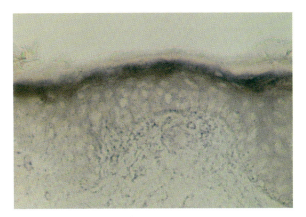

(a)

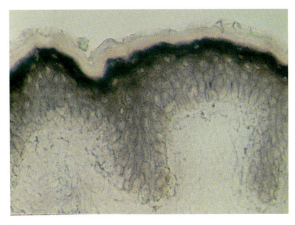

(b)

Figure 7.2

Enzyme cytochemical reactions for glucose-6-phosphate dehydrogenase. (a) Before irradiation with UVE; (b) after irradiation. Note that the reaction product is denser and distributed more widely in the epidermis.

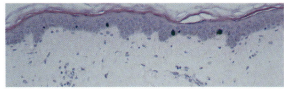

(a)

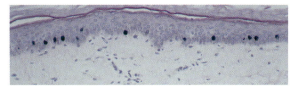

(b)

Figure 7.3

Autoradiographs after exposure of skin to tritiated thymidine to show cells in DNA synthesis (a) from non-exposed skin; (b) from exposed skin. The epidermis is thicker and there are more labelled cells on the basal layer in the exposed skin.

Epidermal dysplasia

Even apparently clinically normal but chronically sun-exposed skin shows a series of histological alterations to the epidermal structure. These minor changes, detectable histologically but not necessarily clinically, are collectively referred to as minimal dysplasia (or photodysplasia). The changes observed include minor degrees of abnormality in cell and nuclear size, shape and staining reaction[1] (Figure 7.1) as well as in cytochemical profile.[2] An example of the latter is the increased glucose-6-phosphate dehydrogenase activity in the upper part of the epidermis in the exposed skin (Figure 7.2). Changes also occur in the succinic dehydrogenase and lactic dehydrogenase activities. The alterations in enzymic activities are quantified by employing a microdensitometer to measure the densities of the reaction products in tissue sections. We proposed that the cytochemical changes be used as the basis of a model of photodamage.

The minor structural changes are accompanied by an increase in the rate of epidermal cell proliferation as evidenced by the increase in the number of basal keratinocytes that incorporate tritiated thymidine after injection[3] or after short-term in vitro incubation. These may be quantified by counting the numbers of epidermal cells that become

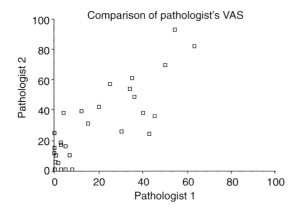

Figure 7.4

Dysplasia scores on visual analogue scale score by two pathologists. There is a good relationship between the two sets of scores.

autoradiographically labelled (labelling index when expressed as a percentage of the total number of basal cells) (Figure 7.3). The labelling index is not a parameter which is difficult to measure but as with other estimates of epidermal cell production it is not sufficiently sensitive to use as an indicator of the severity of photodamage. We have also attempted to quantify the degree of photodysplasia present by assessing the amount (and type) of DNA present in the nuclei of the epidermal cells using a fluorescence-activated cell-sorting device (FACS analysis). Results suggest that this may be a useful approach to the assessment of photodamage, but there are still many technical difficulties to be ironed out.

In one study we attempted to derive a dysplasia index by using a series of histometric parameters derived from an image analysis technique, but are sad to relate that the most reproducible method of assessing the degree of photodysplasia present is still to recruit the services of an experienced dermatopathologist.[4] By employing a visual analogue scale and marking the severity of the dysplasia observed on a 0–10 cm line, a 'semi-subjective quantitative' estimate of the degree of dysplasia present is obtained. Some extra precision may be attainable with the use of an electronic digital visual analogue scale meter. The microscopist moves a lever along a 10-cm long slot and a meter records the position on a digital display. This primitive and potentially observer-biased method has proved satisfactorily reproducible both between observers and when used by a single observer (Figure 7.4). Clearly this technique will be superseded in the not-too-distant future by some method less sensitive to observer bias.

Other epidermal changes

Persistently exposed skin has a thicker and more irregular epidermis than skin from the same site that has not experienced photodamage. The degree of epidermal thickening will depend inter alia on the cumulated amount of photodamage sustained, but is not ideal as a measure of photodamage as the thickness not only records chronic photodamage but also reflects more recent damage from ultraviolet irradiation (UVR). Another confounding problem is that after extreme photodamage the epidermis seems to 'give up the ghost' and instead of being thickened becomes atrophied. The stratum corneum shows no consistent microscopic change in photodamaged skin compared with protected skin, but photodamaged skin clinically has a perceptibly altered surface texture. Clearly the presence of wrinkles and lines, warty excrescences and scaling patches would suggest that the surface texture of photodamaged skin is rougher than normal. At a higher level of magnification, however, it was observed that the skin surface is in fact flatter in photodamaged skin than in non-exposed intrinsically aged skin, whose surface appears somewhat rougher than in younger groups.[5] The results of these studies performed using skin surface replicas and a surface contour

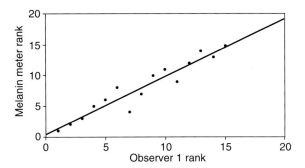

Figure 7.5
Graph to show relationship between the degree of pigmentation as measured by a melanin meter and the amount of melanin present in surface corneocytes as determined by an image analysis method.

tracing device known as a profilometer are at variance with data generated by the Philadelphia group. The differences between the two groups are in all probability explained primarily by differences in the methodology used as well as by differences in the levels of magnification discussed.

Pigmentary changes

Chronic photodamage results in flat brown macules on the backs of the hands, the dorsal surfaces of the forearms and sides of the face. These lesions have come to be known senile lentigines or more colloquially as 'liver spots' in the United Kingdom, or more aptly and colourfully by the French as *'les medallions de cimitière'* and are greatly disliked by the public as they are a real cosmetic nuisance. A better name for them would be solar lentigines. Although they appear to be single entity, careful study by several groups has shown that the same clinical appearance hides seborrhoeic warts, solar keratoses and even lentigo maligna as well as simple lentigo (see Chapter 3). Treatments for these lesions are many and various, but none is completely satisfactory. Some patients are helped by topical tretinoin[6] and presumably by other topical retinoids as well. Others are improved by the older monobenzyl ether of hydroquinone and yet others by 20% azelaic acid either alone or in combination with hydroquinone and/or topical retinoids. The rate of improvement due to the above drugs and other newer agents that are being introduced can be checked by the use of instruments specifically designed to measure skin colour. Two main types of instrument are available commercially. Both are capable of yielding objective and accurate data and are sufficiently sensitive to record small changes in the depth of skin pigmentation. The first of these is the Chromameter (Minolta), which measures colour by an electronic matching process in which colour is assigned co-ordinates in a three-dimensional colour space analysis[7] providing three parameters (the L a. b. system where L = lightness, a = red–green and b = blue–yellow). This instrument was used by the Ann Arbor group to help assess the efficacy of topical tretinoin in the treatment of these brown spots.[6] The other instrument that may be used is the Melanin Meter or the Mexameter (Courage, Khazaka), which employs the dedicated reflectance spectrophotometric principle and which was originally described by Diffey and Farr.[8] The Cardiff group have developed the device into a portable hand-held instrument[9] (Figure 7.5) and used this to measure the effects of several depigmenting agents on senile lentigines in the cortext of clinical trials.

There are other skin colour changes that cause cosmetic distress in photodamage in addition to senile lentigines. The first of these is the muddy or sallow yellow-brown discoloration seen in some severely photodamaged subjects in areas of marked solar elastotic degenerative change (Figure 7.6); this is known sometimes as 'citrine skin'.

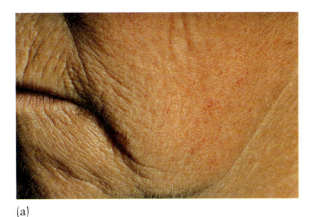 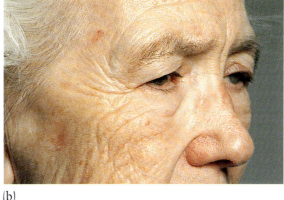

(a) (b)

Figure 7.6

Yellowish skin due to chronic photodamage.

A further colour alteration noted in some sun-damaged subjects is the redness of the cheeks that accompanies the telangiectasia and is mistakenly taken as a sign of 'rude good health' (Figure 7.7). It is in fact 'weathering' and is more often seen in blue-eyed individuals who have Celtic ancestry. There is a strong resemblance between the 'weathering' and the early stages of rosacea—so much so in fact that one is driven to ask whether in fact they are the same condition. Measurements of these changes are possible, but difficult. The erythema of the cheeks can be assessed by either the chromameter or a reflectance spectrophotometer device known as the erythema meter (incorporated into a device known as the Mexameter). Unfortunately, the redness tends to be patchy, making exact placement of the probe critical if serial measurement is going to be used as a measure of disease progress. The sallowness is even more difficult to characterize and evaluate instrumentally. Studies by the Cardiff group using a very sensitive scanning spectrophotometer[10] have been partially successful in producing a reproducible measurement and have identified correlations between the L.a.b. parameters and the elastic tissue content in the upper dermis in photodamaged skin as determined by the image analysis technique. The slope of the line at best fit tended towards the yellow parameter.

Blood flow changes

The degree of redness is a very poor reflection of the rate of blood flow per unit volume of tissue. The reasons for this are that the degree of redness is affected by the degree of skin pigmentation and the thickness of tissue between the vasculature and the skin surface. In addition, blood pooling in dilated vessels can produce redness without there being any increase in the rate of blood flow. This is the situation in rosacea, for example. Blood flow to the skin decreases in intrinsic aging and probably also does so in skin affected by chronic photodamage as well, though there are fewer reliable data for this. Whatever else, topical retinoids cause an increase in the blood flow to the treated site and measures of this have been used for monitoring the progress of the disorder when treated by

114   Photodamaged Skin: Clinical Signs, Causes and Management

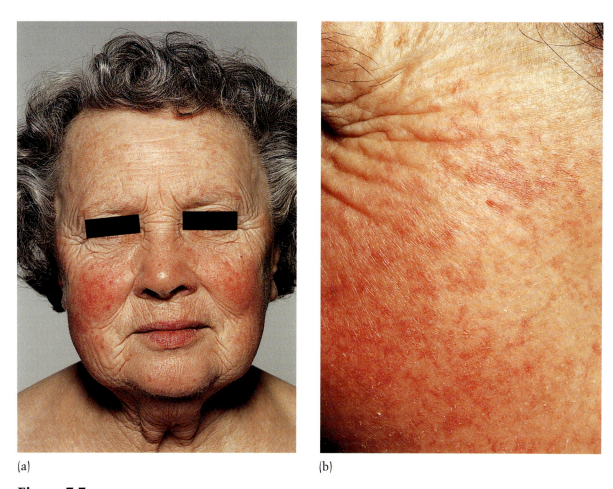

(a) (b)

Figure 7.7
Red cheeks with telangiectasia due to chronic photodamage.

retinoids.[11] The most convenient and most sensitive technique suitable for the assessment of skin blood flow is the laser Doppler flowmeter technique.[12] This depends on the sum total movement of red blood cells in the capillary vasculature in the cubic millimetre of tissue beneath the probe. The device is not difficult to use and the cost, although high, is certainly within reach of most dermatology departments. A new 'scanning' laser Doppler device has been introduced which allows imaging in the horizontal dimension on the basis of skin blood flow.

Measures of solar elastosis

Topical retinoids and other newer types of drug in development accelerate removal of elastotic degenerate material and stimulate the synthesis of new dermal connective tissue in situ. To assess the efficacy of these agents and to record the degree of elastosis present some objective measure(s) is (are) required. Measurements of the degree of elastosis from skin biopsies are certainly possible and indeed have been made to assess whether the use of sunscreens over prolonged periods causes

The measurement of photodamage

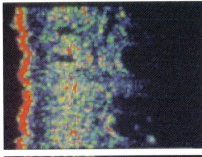

Sun exposed
Skin: 1.22mm
SENEB: 0.41mm
(34%)

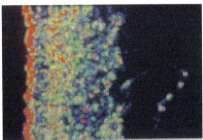

Sun protected
Skin: 1.31mm
SENEB: 0.28mm
(21%)

Figure 7.8

B-scan ultrasound to show echolucent area subepidermally representing solar elastotic change. Note that the echolucent band is broader in the sun exposed image compared with the image from sun-protected skin. (With grateful thanks to Dr Jean-Luc Leveque, L'Oreal, Paris.)

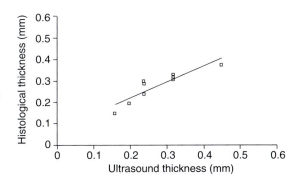

Figure 7.9

Graph to show relationship between the amount of elastotic degenerative change determined by the image analysis method and the thickness of solar elastotic tissue supepidermally as determined by A-scan ultrasound.

reduction in the degree of elastosis present.[13] Essentially an image analysis technique needs to be employed in which the elastotic material is heavily stained by one of the stains used histologically such as Halmis' stain or elastic van Gieson and then 'detected' and quantified in an image analysis microscope. An alternative approach is to measure the mean depth of the elastic-staining material below the epidermis in the sections examined. The main difficulty with these techniques is the need to assume that the degree of elastosis of the area of skin in question is adequately represented by the amount of solar elastosis in the small piece of skin removed by the biopsy procedure. There are few data available that can assure us as to the reliability of these measurements, although inspection of biopsies suggests that the elastotic degenerative process is not focal or very variable and this measurement technique is capable of yielding reliable data.

For obvious reasons, if serial measurements are to be made, non-invasive measures are preferable. The most direct and possibly the most reliable of these is the measurement of the depth to which the elastotic change extends within the skin by high-resolution ultrasound. My own preference has been to use pulsed A-scan ultrasound,[14] but several groups have employed the B-scan imaging mode successfully.[15] The ability to measure the degree of elastosis depends on the differing acoustic properties of elastotic dermis compared with normal fibrous dermis. The elastotic dermis is echolucent because of the loss of the normal fibrillar structure, when compared with the normal fibrous dermis, which is echogenic. The echolucent elastotic dermis is easily distinguished from the echogenic normal dermis (Figure 7.8) and its width can be measured without difficulty. We have shown that there is a strong relationship between the width of the echolucent band and the amount of elastosis determined histometrically from biopsy samples[16] (Figure 7.9). The ultrasound technique is simple, painless, completely safe and relatively quick. Unfortunately, the outlay cost of ultrasound equipment is significant, although when spread over a large number of observations the cost of individual readings will be very small.

Measurement of the mechanical properties of chronically exposed and photodamaged skin is one other way of assessing solar elastotic degenerative change. There is no doubt that the mechanical responses of photodamaged skin are markedly altered compared with non-exposed skin and that these changes can be detected and measured using any of the various devices that have been described for the investigation of skin[17] (see Chapters 2 and 5). A suction device known as the Cutometer[18] has proved quite helpful in characterizing photodamaged skin. This relies on measurement of the height of a bubble of skin 'sucked' through a variably sized port. Pierard and co-workers have described a potentially important parameter termed the 'cutaneous extrinsic aging score' derived from data obtained using the Cutometer, which is proposed as a measure of solar elastosis. Overall a decrease in elasticity, extensibility and maximum deformation is typical of photodamaged skin. Other devices used to measure the mechanical characteristics of photodamaged skin include the twistometer,[19] the linear uniaxial extensometer[20] and the levarometer.[21] While of research interest, these various techniques have variables which are difficult to control, such as the 'stress history' of the part examined and the ambient environmental conditions, and the data are often difficult to interpret.

The altered mechanical properties of solar elastotic dermis are responsible for many of the lines and wrinkles on sun-exposed skin, including the so-called crow's-feet at the sides of the eyes. The presence of these crow's feet at the lateral margins of the orbits is a major cause of cosmetic discomfort and their extent has been used as measure of the degree of photodamage present (Figure 7.10). Many of

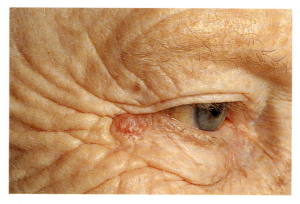

Figure 7.10

Crow's-feet at the lateral margin of the orbit. There is also a basal cell carcinoma at the commissure.

the multicentre studies of 0.05% tretinoin for the treatment of chronic photodamage assessed the severity of the crow's-feet sign by taking silicone rubber impressions from the lateral orbital site in a commendably standardized way, sending them to a central laboratory in Philadelphia and then measuring the surface contour of the impressions optically using an image analysis device. The scans were performed in two directions – horizontally and laterally, or 'north–south' and 'east–west', as the authors described them. The replicas were assessed blind to avoid any bias. These studies successfully demonstrated the efficacy of the topical tretinoin and were quite supportive of the clinical findings.

Clinical methods

So far we have dealt with measurement of the effects of persistent sun exposure on different aspects of skin structure and function using different instruments and techniques, and have not discussed more direct clinical measurements. They are of course central to the clinical issue, but despite the lack of devices and complicated technology are actually quite difficult to carry out reproducibly and with a sufficient degree of sensitivity to make the measures discriminating. All the published studies of the efficacy of topical retinoids for chronic photodamage have used clinical scores as the main efficacy variables, as well as a range of other techniques to support the clinical findings.

The particular physical signs evaluated depend on the specific therapeutic question being asked and will depend on the agent being used, as not all agents will necessarily have the same spectrum of effects. Amongst the most frequently used clinical parameters of photoaging used are 'fine lines', dyspigmentation, skin roughness, yellowish discoloration and the rosy red appearance of the cheeks that appears after treatment with topical retinoids. 'Global' evaluations are also used in which the clinician gives an overall view of the severity of the photodamage. As can be expected, categorizing the severity of any of these parameters in an objective, sensitive and reproducible way is not easy. It is important to categorize the severity numerically so as to be able to pool data and determine the statistical significances of any differences found. In most studies short ordinal scales are used in which the severity of the particular physical sign in question is given as 1, 2, 3 or 4 to match the descriptive terms such as mild, marked, severe and very severe. Sometimes the scale is expanded by giving half-points, or extended up to 6 or more. Certainly, the longer the scale, the greater the potential sensitivity. The major problem of ordinal scales of this type is that they are non-equal-interval in type—i.e. the gap between 1 and 2 in severity is not necessarily the same as between 3 and 4 or between 4 and 5. The relatively limited number of choices when using a short ordinal scale results in lack of reproducibility and sensitivity.

An alternative to use of a short non-equal-interval ordinal scale is a visual analogue scale (VAS). In this system the severity is scored on a 10-cm scale by placing a cross in pencil on a 10-cm-long line previously drawn or printed. This simple manoeuvre converts the scoring system into a more sensitive technique just by virtue of the fact that the score can be anywhere between 0 and 10 and is not forced artificially into one of a very few categories. This VAS method also tends to be more reproducible. To save making a mark on a line and then having to measure it subsequently, we have devised a system based on an electronic meter with a liquid crystal display digital read-out.

The use of a graded series of photographs showing patients with increasing degrees of photodamage has been described by Griffiths et al.[22] Each of the five grades had two photographs (en face and 45° oblique) and allowed the clinicians to grade their patients on a nine-point scale by comparing them to the photographs. This system was shown to have good interobserver agreement and appears to be a simple, useful, inexpensive way of improving the reproducibility of clinical evaluations.

Photographic techniques

Using serial photographs to assess progress in any dermatological disorder appears deceptively easy. In photodamage it is even more difficult than in inflammatory skin diseases such as acne, psoriasis or atopic dermatitis. Small differences in camera–subject alignments and distance, in lighting, in background, in film speed or photographic emulsion sensitivity and in development methods can result in photographs which seem to show a dramatic difference even though they were taken a few minutes apart! Even when the photographic and development technique has been extraordinarily fastidious the question as to how to evaluate the photographs without bias creeping in and how to employ some kind of objective and quantative measure from the photographic image remains.

In recent years these difficulties in the use of photographic assessments have been widely appreciated. Those pharmaceutical companies with topical retinoids for use in photodamage have been careful to employ impeccable photographic techniques as part of their investigations so that the accusation that the photographic evidence is not trustworthy can no longer be made. One study in which topical isotretinoin was assessed for the treatment of photodamage stands out as a model for the use of objective photographic technique.[23] In this trial the subjects were photographed in a rigorous standardized protocol. The 'before' and 'after' photographs were then projected onto two screens side by side by two projectors so that the choice of which screen the befores and after of each pair were projected onto was always made at random. The two screens were viewed by five dermatologists who did not know the randomization code and had to assess each of the photographs for particular clinical features of photodamage. The study demonstrated unequivocally that the topical retinoid employed had a significantly superior therapeutic effect compared with the placebo cream used as comparator.

Conclusion

Clinical measurements are now essential to the practice of medicine. Dermatology has been late in recognizing this, but now embraces objective and quantitative techniques as part of the assessment of all new drugs for the treatment of skin disease, as well as using these measurement techniques in the daily care of patients. Photoaging requires special care in its quantification and the methods described should be of assistance for this purpose.

References

1. Marks R, The pathology of chronic solar damage and the effects of topical tretinoin. *J Dermatol Treat* (1996) **7**(suppl 2): 513–17.
2. Pearse AD, Marks R, Response of human skin to ultraviolet radiation; dissociation of erythema and metabolic changes following sunscreen protection. *J Invest Dermatol* (1983) **80**: 191–4.
3. Pearse AD, Marks R, Actinic keratoses and the epidermis on which they arise. *Br J Dermatol* (1977) **96**: 45–50.
4. Barton SP, Pearse AD, Marks R, Derivation of a dysplasia index for epidermal neoplasia. *Dermatology* (1992) **185**: 190–5.
5. Edwards CE, Heggie RH, Marks R, A study of differences in surface roughness between exposed and unexposed skin with age. (In Press).
6. Griffiths CEM, Goldfarb MT, Finkel LJ et al, Topical tretinoin (retinoic acid) treatment of hyperpigmented lesions associated with photoaging in Chinese and Japanese patients: a vehicle controlled trial. *J Am Acad Dermatol* (1994) **30**: 76–84.
7. Weatherall IL, Coombs BD, Skin colour measurements in terms of CIELAB colour space values. *J Invest Dermatol* (1992) **7**: 217–25.
8. Farr PM, Diffey BL, Quantitative studies on cutaneous erythema induced by ultraviolet radiation. *Br J Dermatol* (1984) **111**: 673–82.
9. Pearse AD, Edwards C, Hill S, Marks R, Portable erythema meter and its application to use in human skin. *Int J Cos Sci* (1990) **12**: 63–70.
10. Nishimori Y, Pearse AD, Edwards C et al, Elastotic degenerative change and yellowish discolouration in photoaged skin. *Skin Res and Tech* (1998) **4**: 79–82.
11. Effency I, Weltfriend S, Patil S, Maibach HI, Differential irritant skin responses to topical retinoic acid and sodium lauryl sulphate: alone and in crossover design. *Br J Dermatol* (1996) **134**: 424–30.

12. Nilsson GE, Tenland T, Oberg PA, A new instrument for continuous measurement of tissue blood flow by light beating spectroscopy. *IEEE Trans Biomed Eng* (1980) **BME-27**: 12–19.
13. Boyd AS, Naylor M, Cameron G et al, The effects of chronic sunscreen use on histologic changes in dermatoheliosis. *J Am Acad Dermatol* (1995) **33**: 941–6.
14. Tan CY, Statham B, Marks R, Payne PA, Skin thickness measurement by pulsed ultrasound: its reproducibility, validation and variability. *Br J Dermatol* (1982) **106**: 657–67.
15. Serup J, High frequency ultrasound examination of aged skin: intrinsic, actinic and gravitational aging, including new concepts of stasis dermatitis and by ulcer. In: J Léveque (ed.) *Aging Skin. Properties and Functional Changes*. Marcel Dekker: New York, 1993, pp. 69.
16. Edwards C, Al-Aboosi MM, Marks R, The use of A-scan ultrasound in the diagnosis and measurement of small skin tumours. *Br J Dermatol* (1989) **121**: 297–304.
17. Serup J, Jemec GBE (eds), *Handbook of Non invasive Methods and the Skin*. CRC Press: Baton Rouge, 1995.
18. Couturaud V, Coutable J, Khajat A, Skin biomechanical properties: in vivo evaluation of influence of age and body site by a non invasive method. *Skin Res and Tech* (1995) **1**: 68–73.
19. Agache P, Mooneur C, Leveque JL, de Rigal J, Mechanical properties and Young's modulus of human skin in vivo. *Arch Dermatol Res* (1980) **269**: 221–32.
20. Gunner CW, Hutton WC, Berlin TE. The mechanical properties of skin in vivo – a portable hand held extensometer. *Br J Dermatol* (1979) **100**: 161–3.
21. Dikstein S, Hartzshtark A, In vivo measurement of some elastic properties of human skin. In: Marks R, Payne PA (eds), *Bioengineering and the Skin*. MTP Press: Lancaster, pp. 45–53.
22. Griffiths CEM, Wang TS, Hamilton TA et al, A photonumeric scale of the assessment of cutaneous photodamage. *Arch Dermatol* (1992) **128**: 347–51.
23. Armstrong RB, Lesiewicz J, Jarvey G et al, Clinical panel assessment of photodamaged skin treated with isotretinoin using photographs. *Arch Dermatol* (1992) **128**: 352–6.

8 The treatment of skin photoaging

Medical therapy

Topical retinoids

Despite the existence of a large number of synthetic retinoids with biological activity, clinical data on their topical use for photodamage therapy are available for only a few, including all-*trans*-retinoic acid (tretinoin), the 13-*cis*-isomer of retinoic acid (isotretinoin) and retinaldehyde (retinal). A few others, including esters of retinoic acid, are being studied.

Tretinoin (all-trans-retinoic acid)

Photoaging. A large number of double-blind vehicle-controlled studies have shown that topically applied tretinoin is an effective treatment of photodamage in humans. Kligman et al[1] provided the first demonstration that tretinoin can partially reverse photodamage in an unblinded vehicle-controlled study in Caucasians. They observed clinical, histological and physiological changes in facial and forearm skin treated with 0.05% tretinoin cream (Retin A) twice daily for 3 months, which indicated partial reversal of much of the photodamage induced by ultraviolet light. A subsequent double-blind vehicle-controlled study involving 30 Caucasian subjects from ages 35 to 70 with unspecified degrees of photodamage used 0.1% cream on their faces and forearms for 4 months.[2] All patients who used tretinoin cream showed statistically significant improvement in photoaging on their faces and forearms compared with those who applied vehicle. Topical tretinoin treatment improved coarse and fine wrinkling, hyperpigmentation and roughness, and induced an increase in pinkness ('rosy glow'). Histological changes were also observed in treated skin, including epidermal hyperplasia, stratum corneum compaction, reduced melanocytic hypertrophy and increased vascularity in the papillary dermis. These observations were confirmed by ultrastructural analysis, which in addition demonstrated increased collagen formation, hyperactive fibroblasts and more-normal-appearing elastic tissue.[3] The most common side-effect during the treatment was a tretinoin-induced dermatitis associated with xerosis, peeling and subjective irritation and persistent mild erythema. These authors suggested that topical retinoids might exert influences in intrinsically aged skin similar to those seen in photodamage. They also commented that no evidence was found to support a role for retinoid-induced irritation or oedema as in the reduction of wrinkling. Further studies confirmed and extended these findings.[4,5] Fine lines, wrinkles, texture, pigmentary blotchiness and sallowness were significantly improved with tretinoin therapy. Furthermore, the clinical improvement was confirmed by an objective method of optical profilometry[6] based on digital image-processing of silicone rubber casts obtained from the crow's feet area. This technique indicated that the skin was smoother and less wrinkled in the tretinoin-treated group than in the vehicle control group.[5]

Additional larger studies were performed using a newer formulation of tretinoin emollient cream at 0.05% and 0.01% concentrations.[7] Two hundred and fifty-one Caucasian subjects with mild to moderate photodamage were treated with the tretinoin emollient cream or the vehicle for 6 months. Clinical grading showed a greater reduction in mean overall severity over the treatment period in the group of subjects who applied 0.05% tretinoin emollient cream than in subjects on tretinoin 0.01%, suggesting a dose-related response. Significant improvement was observed only for the 0.05% tretinoin group compared with the vehicle group. The average reduction of the specific symptoms (27.1 per cent for fine wrinkling, 29.3 per cent for roughness and 37 per cent for mottled hyperpigmentation) was significantly better in subjects treated with 0.05% tretinoin cream than in patients applying the 0.01% tretinoin cream or the control vehicle. Histological results also demonstrated dose-related changes for epidermal melanin content. However, no changes were noted in the papillary dermis thickness, the presence of mucin, elastosis, collagen regeneration, perivascular inflammation and reversal of keratinocyte atypia. Another large study using tretinoin emollient cream confirmed these findings.[8] In all these studies, the most common side-effects included mild erythema, peeling, burning and stinging. These reactions were mild to moderate, rarely leading to discontinuation of treatment. They decreased gradually during therapy, but continued in many patients over the 6-month treatment period. These side-effects either resolved spontaneously or were considerably lessened by emollient use.

The value of further long-term tretinoin treatment for photodamage was also evaluated. Subjects using 0.05% tretinoin emollient cream for a total of 12 months retained their improvement during the second 6 months with a slope of improvement appearing to plateau.[9] Side-effects continued to be present but with decreased frequency. Those subjects who continued the daily use of 0.05% tretinoin emollient cream for an additional 6 months (12–18 months) were randomized into three groups: three applications per week versus one application per week versus discontinuation of treatment. At the end of this evaluation period, 63 per cent and 64 per cent of the patients who used 0.05% tretinoin emollient cream once or three times a week, respectively, maintained the improvement obtained after 12 months of continuous treatment. Few subjects achieved further improvement during the last 6 months. Of the patients 53 per cent discontinued treatment after 12 months of once a day use of 0.05% tretinoin emollient cream were noted to have regressed.

A few long-term studies are available. In one of them, 27 patients were treated with tretinoin emollient cream for up to 18 months, followed by further treatment with a 0.01% concentration for up to 15 months longer, and finally by a 19-month daily treatment with tretinoin cream 0.025 or 0.05%. Histological studies of the skin of these patients treated for up to 4 years demonstrated a slight decrease in epidermal thickness between 12 months and 4 years. However, the increase in the granular layer thickness, the reduction in the epidermal melanin content and the stratum corneum compaction remained unchanged.[10]

Intrinsic aging. The effects of tretinoin are not limited to photoaging. In six patients, aged 68–79 years who applied 0.025% tretinoin cream on the inner aspect of one thigh and vehicle cream to the opposite side once daily for 9 months, tretinoin induced only a modest clinical improvement. The tretinoin-treated skin was less wrinkled, less scaly, a little firmer and had a pink hue. In contrast, there was a marked histological improvement in the involutional structural changes of 'intrinsically' aged human skin. Tretinoin treatment produced a marked increase in the viable epidermal thickness and resulted in a more undulating dermoepidermal junction with prominent rete ridges. Ultrastructural changes at the dermoepidermal junction included the development of anchoring fibrils. In the dermis, angiogenesis was particularly noteworthy as well as new elastic fibres and increases in glycosaminoglycan deposition. All these morphological observations demonstrate that topical tretinoin substantially altered the involutional structural changes in intrinsically aged protected skin and that the magnitude of these changes may be even greater than those described for photodamaged skin.[11]

These in vivo observations are confirmed by an in vitro study demonstrating in organ culture that the effect of tretinoin on both sun-exposed and non-sun-exposed skin in adults produced identical responses in both types of skin. Tretinoin improved the histological appearance of the epidermis and dermis in adult skin cultures.

Guidelines for the use of topical tretinoin. Tretinoin treatment must be individualized. First, it is most important to choose the appropriate formulation in relation to the potential skin sensitivity of the patient. In patients with severe photodamage and low skin sensitivity, large pores and oily skin, such as darker, thick-skinned, Mediterranean patients, a 0.1% tretinoin preparation may represent a good therapeutic option. Several studies suggest that a 0.1% preparation may represent a better therapeutic approach for treatment of the individual with severely photoaged skin. In most patients, a 0.05% tretinoin preparation represents the most reasonable starting concentration. In patients with great skin sensitivity, initiating therapy with a concentration lower than 0.05% may be preferable to minimize irritation at the beginning, gradually increasing the concentration to reach standard regimens. Patients with the greatest skin sensitivity include fair-skinned, freckled, blue-eyed patients (phototype I), patients who have 'sensitive' skin, flusher-blushers, heavy users of cosmetics and cleansers, and subjects with prior skin disorders such as rosacea or seborrhoeic dermatitis.[12]

In a recent double-blind, vehicle-controlled comparative study, 0.1% and 0.025% tretinoin creams produced similar clinical and histological changes in patients with photoaging. After 48 weeks, both creams produced significant epidermal thickening (by 30 per cent and 28 per cent respectively). Irritant side-effects were statistically greater with 0.1% tretinoin than with 0.025% tretinoin. This lack of correspondence between clinical improvement and irritation suggests that mechanisms other than irritation dominate tretinoin-induced repair of photoaging in humans. Furthermore, this study dispels the previous belief that the higher the active concentration used in the treatment of photoaging, the greater and faster the subsequent improvement.[13]

Tretinoin should be used as above and patients must become active partners in the treatment programme.[12] The initial visit must include detailed information about the topical preparation, its side-effects and the time course of improvement. Poorly informed patients will soon abandon therapy because of discomfort or because of overexpectation. The following points should be emphasized before initiation of therapy.

The tretinoin preparation must be applied on the skin after washing with a mild soap and patting the skin dry. Patients are instructed to apply an amount of cream that thinly covers the entire face, excluding the eyelids and the corners of the mouth. The drug can be used around the eyes and mouth, where wrinkles are very common, but the patient should be informed that transient stinging and burning will occur and that this is harmless. This should be the last act of the day.[12] For the face, on average, a 20-g tube should last almost 6 weeks, and a 45-g tube should last approximately 3 months, varying somewhat depending on the area of the face being treated.[9]

In patients with sensitive skin, the applications can be performed every other day from initiation of treatment or as soon as excessive irritation occurs. Most patients can regulate treatment by adjusting the dose and frequency of application. All patients must be informed that skin discomfort will occur during the initial phase of treatment, sometimes leading to a decrease in the frequency of application, but that it will be possible to end up with one daily application after the accommodation phase.

The patients should be informed that this topical treatment is not a substitute for facelifts, since overexpectation leads to profound disappointment. They should know that not all signs of photodamage to skin respond to this treatment and that the clinical benefits are slow and may not be apparent for months. They must be told that tretinoin can reverse some of the clinical features of photodamage but is also a prophylactic agent to prevent and slow the progression of photoaging. Although long-term tretinoin treatments are not standardized, the patients must be informed that a maintenance treatment will be required to retain the clinical improvement.

Finally, the physician must emphasize that the tretinoin therapy is the core of a larger treatment programme to improve and/or prevent the damaging cutaneous effects of chronic sun exposure. Supplementary treatment, including moisturizers to control the side-effects of topical retinoid therapy and broad-spectrum sunscreens, are a must for these patients. Moisturizers should be carefully chosen for their good tolerability.[12] They should not be used at the same time as the topical retinoid. Morning application every day after washing the face should be recommended and a few studies demonstrate that this strategy effectively reduces the skin dryness induced by topical retinoids. The broad-spectrum sunscreens are necessary to counteract the partial loss of sun protection due to retinoid-induced thinning of the stratum corneum and to prevent further skin photodamage.

Mechanisms of action. Retinoids exert pleiotropic effects by modulating gene transcription after interacting with cytoplasmic binding proteins and binding to nuclear receptors. Retinoic acid induces a characteristic set of biochemical and histological alterations leading to clinical improvement when applied to photodamaged skin. It is likely that many of these effects are mediated by nucleic acid receptors acting through retinoic acid response elements located in the regulatory regions of target genes.

After topical application of all-*trans*-retinoic acid (RA), approximately 50 per cent remains in the all-*trans*-form.[14] The remaining 50 per cent is converted within the epidermis and probably the dermis to 13-*cis*-, 9-*cis*- and 4-hydroxyretinoic acid. RA and its isomers bind to specific nuclear receptors, members of the steroid/thyroid hormone nuclear receptor superfamily which function as ligand-dependent transcription factors.

Nuclear retinoic acid receptors comprise two families each encoded by three genes. The nuclear retinoic acid receptor family, called RAR, which comprises three forms (RAR-α, -β, -γ) was the first to be described.[15] These RARs, expressed as isoforms generated by the use of multiple transcriptional start sites and/or alternative splicing, bind and are activated by all-*trans*-retinoic acid. A second family of nuclear receptors termed retinoid X receptors also consists of three members,

RXR-α, RXR-β, RXR-γ, and was isolated more recently. RXRs are activated by 9-*cis*-RA. 9-*cis*-RA binds to both RARs and RXRs with similar high affinity, whereas all-*trans*-RA binds with high affinity to RARs but only very weakly to RXRs. RARs form heterodimers with RXRs. In human epidermis and cultured keratinocytes, Western and Northern analysis demonstrates that the constitutive levels of RAR-α and -β mRNA and proteins are very low or not detectable, whereas those of RAR-γ are high, representing 87 per cent of RAR protein.[16-18] Both isoforms of RAR-γ, RAR-γ1 and RAR-γ2, are detectable, with RAR-γ1 being the more strongly expressed.[17] Protein levels of RXRs are five times greater than those of RARs.[16] RXR-α represents 90 per cent of RXR protein expressed in human skin. No RXR-β or RXR-γ can be detected by Western blot.[19] These relative RXR protein levels mirror their relative mRNA levels in human skin. Thus, the two predominant forms of retinoic acid and retinoid X receptors in human skin are RAR-γ and RXR-α.[20]

In normal human keratinocytes, endogenous RAR/RXR heterodimers are the major function forms regulating retinoid-responsive elements in target genes.[21] Furthermore, interaction among RXRs is much lower than that between RAR and RXR.[21] These recent findings demonstrate that the retinoid receptor-mediated nuclear pathway is more complex than previously thought, and the question of the receptor-specificity of retinoids should be re-examined in the light of these observations. Synthetic retinoids able independently to trigger the RXR homodimer- and RAR/RXR heterodimer-mediated pathways are already available and are of great potential for therapeutic use.

Isotretinoin (13-CIS-retinoic acid)

In the UVB-irradiated hairless mouse model, isotretinoin is active in inducing structural modifications at the dermal level and in wrinkle effacement. A double-blind, vehicle-controlled clinical trial using isotretinoin 0.05% cream for 12 weeks followed by isotretinoin 0.1% cream during the next 24 weeks, applied once nightly in 776 patients with mild to moderate photodamage, demonstrated that isotretinoin resulted in statistically significant improvement in overall appearance, fine wrinkling, discrete pigmentation, sallowness and texture. Fewer than 5 per cent of the patients experienced severe intolerance reactions and few patients withdrew from the study because of local irritation. These results indicate that topical isotretinoin treatment improves some of the signs of cutaneous photodamage.[22]

Retinaldehyde

Human keratinocytes transform retinol into retinaldehyde and then into retinoic acid by two enzymatic steps involving dehydrogenases. Thus, retinaldehyde is an interesting retinoic acid precursor for topical use because it by-passes the rate-limiting step of retinol oxidation into retinoic acid. Furthermore, differentiating keratinocytes are able to convert retinaldehyde into RA at a higher rate than are non-differentiated keratinocytes. Only keratinocytes capable of retinaldehyde oxidation at a pertinent stage of differentiation would generate RA, resulting in a more controlled RA delivery and putatively weaker side-effects as compared with direct application of RA or synthetic analogues. Topical retinaldehyde is well tolerated on human skin and has biological activity (induction of CRABP2 protein and mRNA expression, increased epidermal thickness, keratin-14 expression and keratinocyte proliferation).

Long-term application (6 months) of a cream containing 0.05% retinaldehyde is well tolerated and induced significant beneficial effects on the appearance of skin in 32 female patients with mild to moderate photoaging. The results, evaluated by both clinical and instrumental assessment techniques, showed an improvement of the clinical features of photoaging with attenuation of the degree of wrinkling, a reduction in facial erythema and improvement in the brightness, smoothness and general comfort of their skin. The cream was well tolerated. Thus, 0.05% retinaldehyde may be of use in the treatment of photodamaged skin.[23]

α-*Hydroxy acids (AHAs)*

Clinical studies

AHAs can be used effectively and safely as peeling agents to improve photoaged skin. AHAs, such as glycolic, lactic and citric acids, are acids that are found naturally occurring in plants and animals. Glycolic acid, one of the most commonly used AHAs, is found in sugar cane. Glycolic acid has been reported to cause epidermolysis when applied to the skin for 3–7 minutes. However, the skin response depends on the glycolic acid concentration, on the pH, on the vehicle, on the duration of contact with the skin and on the amount of free acid delivered to the skin. Thus glycolic acid can be used to evoke a controlled event in the skin that initially results in exfoliation of the superficial layers of the epidermis (desquamation) or deeper (epidermolysis).

Glycolic acid can readily be used as a conventional therapeutic peeling agent. Glycolic acid peel solution may be prepared by dissolving glycolic acid in water and ethanol to make 70%, 50%, 35% and 20% concentrations.[24]

If the acid is left in contact with the skin for more than 10 minutes, deep epidermolysis and penetration to the dermis occur. However, glycolic acid is mainly used as a superficial chemical peeling agent. These 'refresher peels' or 'lunchtime peels' differ from conventional therapeutic peels in that there is little skin reaction (a trace of erythema or irritation which can be concealed with make-up) and patients can go about their regular business without concern. The patient must be cautioned that since glycolic acid will be used to achieve more superficial effects, it is necessary to repeat the procedure at scheduled intervals. Very few studies have been done to assess the efficacy of this procedure. In one double-blind vehicle-controlled study, glycolic acid (50%) or vehicle was applied for 5 minutes to one side of the face, forearms and hands once weekly for 4 weeks in patients with mildly photoaged skin.[25]

A significant improvement was noted on the side treated with glycolic acid, including reduction in rough texture and fine wrinkling, fewer solar keratoses and slight lightening of solar lentigines. Histology confirmed these clinical findings by demonstrating thinning of the stratum corneum, granular layer enhancement, epidermal thickening and increase in collagen thickness in the dermis. In another controlled study, using a different protocol performed in a small number of patients ($n = 12$) showing a moderate degree of photodamage, it was concluded that no specific benefit could be assigned to the use of monthly glycolic acid (70%) refresher peels over a period of 4 months.[26]

Topical moisturizers based on AHAs may be useful in improving photoaged skin. In one study involving 17 subjects with moderate to severe photodamage, patients applied twice daily a lotion containing 25% glycolic (7 subjects), lactic (5) or citric acid (5) to one forearm and a placebo lotion to the opposite forearm for an average of 6 months.[27]

Treatment with AHAs caused an approximate 25 per cent increase in skin thickness. This difference between AHA and vehicle treatment was statistically significant. No significant difference in response among the three AHAs was noted. Histology revealed that this increase in skin thickness was caused by epidermal and papillary dermal thickening without dermal oedema. Another study examined the effect of low (5%) and a higher (12%) concentration on various properties of the facial skin of subjects ranging from 35 to 50 years.[28] Treatment with 12% lactic acid resulted in increased epidermal and dermal firmness and thickness and clinical improvement in skin smoothness and in the appearance of lines and wrinkles. No dermal changes were observed after treatment with 5% lactic acid; however, similar clinical and epidermal changes were noted.

Thus, many studies to date have shown that topical applications of AHAs for periods of a few months induce measurable changes suggestive of reversal of photodamage.[23] Longer-term studies are required to establish the real potential and the true benefit of this treatment.

Other AHAs and/or different formulations need to be tested to achieve greater specificity of action or enhanced potency for greater dermal response.

Mechanism of action

Several AHAs (as well as β-hydroxy and carboxylic acids) in low concentrations stimulate epidermal turnover or cell renewal. Topical ammonium lactate causes an increase in dermal ground substance and increased glycosaminoglycan synthesis, and aggressive glycolic peels significantly increase collagen and dermal ground substance, demonstrating that α-hydroxy acids influence both the epidermis and the dermis. The molecular mechanisms by which AHAs produce these effects are not known. Further ultrastructural studies demonstrate that topical AHAs reduce the number of desmosomes and decrease tonofilament aggregation. In the dermis histochemical stains combined with quantitative morphometry confirm the increase in collagen fibre density in AHA-treated skin.

Treatment of the skin with AHAs leads to mast cell degranulation and increased expression of factor XIIIa transglutaminase by activated dermal dendrocytes. Mast cell degranulation may lead to activation of dermal dendrocytes and increased factor XIIIa transglutaminase expression, via the activation of tumour necrosis factor-α. As the function of intracellular factor XIIIa transglutaminase is unknown, the relation of this finding to improvement of photoaged skin by AHAs is still open to speculation.[29]

Emollients and cosmetics

Aged skin is usually dry. The constant use of moisturizers will help keep the skin hydrated and smooth. The majority of moisturizers, cosmetic or pharmaceutical, are mixtures of oil and water. They are useful adjuvant treatment in the management of dry skin.

Surgical management

Implantable materials

A number of implantable materials useful in the management of facial lines and wrinkles have been developed, including liquid silicone, bovine collagen implant and gelatin matrix implants.[30]

Injectable liquid silicone

Silicone is injected through multiple punctures in microdroplets. Each droplet will induce its own fibroblastic response and result in added augmentation.[31] For this reason, overcorrection must be strictly avoided and undercorrection is the rule. The level at which silicone is injected varies with the depth of lesion in question. Superficial wrinkles should be treated with intradermal

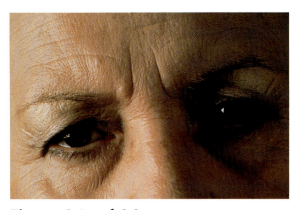 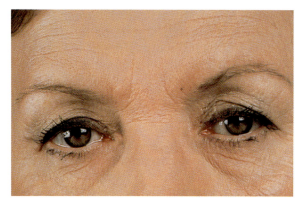

Figures 8.1 and 8.2
Before and after pictures of hylaform implants (Hyaluronic acid) (courtesy of Collagen corporation).

injection, whereas deep, full-thickness contour defects need to be injected at the dermal–fat junction. A risk of the development of 'beading' in a plane above the contour defect is associated with injections which are too superficial. Most facial lines and wrinkles should be augmented gradually over several treatments at monthly or greater intervals. The results are extremely technique-sensitive. Prior training with a qualified clinician before using this material is mandatory.

Side-effects include erythema, swelling and bruising for a few days and temporary beading for a few months at treatment sites, which subsides spontaneously or requires intralesional injections of steroids. Idiosyncratic reactions to silicone, characterized by swelling and erythema, may appear months after injections. They required intralesional corticosteroids and oral antibiotics. Foreign body granulomas have been reported after 'silicone' injections.[31] These problems are due either to impurities and additives present in the injected material or to significant misuse of the material (injection into inappropriate anatomical sites; reckless overcorrection with subsequent lymphatic blockage).

Bovine collagen implants

These implants include solubilized, purified bovine dermal collagen reconstituted in phosphate-buffered saline (Zyderm collagen implant I and II) and cross-linked bovine collagen fibrils (Zyplast collagen implants) to slow the rate of collagenase digestion.[32] Another injected collagen from a Japanese company (Koken) is also available.[30]

Zyderm I or II is indicated for the treatment of superficial fine lines, whereas Zyplast is used for the treatment of deep, coarser lines. Careful massage of the treatment site is performed after injection to blend the interface of the implanted and untreated skin. The duration of correction for active expression lines of the central face is generally around 6 months and supplementary treatment will be required to maintain the correction. A light and electron microscopic evaluation of treated sites demonstrates that Zyderm and Zyplast are identified in the mid- and deep dermis and also intradermally in 60–70 per cent of the samples.[34] The collagen implants are slowly colonized by fibroblasts. Some new collagen deposition was observed associated

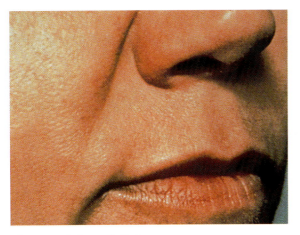 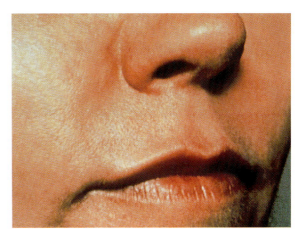

Figures 8.3 and 8.4
Before and after pictures of softform implants, nasolabial folds (expanded polytetrafluoroethylene – EPTFE) (courtesy of Collagen corporation).

with remodelling of Zyplast. These observations suggest that the collagen implants migrate deeper and eventually move to the subcutaneous plane. This movement could explain the loss of correction for 6–9 months that is noted when this implant is used for age-related changes.[34]

A Zyderm test should be performed 1 month prior to initiating treatment, followed by a second skin test on the opposite arm 2 weeks later to further detect sensitization to Zyderm induced by the first test. Allergic reactions include erythema, induration and pruritus at the treatment sites. These reactions may persist for up to 18 months until all the implanted collagen has been digested, but usually subside within 6 months. This immunological reaction is associated with the presence of circulating antibodies to bovine collagen implant. Severe symptoms may require a treatment with antihistamines or with a short course of systemic steroids, but patients should be informed that lowering the inflammatory response may delay the resolution of this allergic reaction. Skin necrosis, usually occurring at only one of the injected sites, may be observed, often in patients who have tolerated previous treatments well. This side-effect may be due either to direct injection into a vessel or to pressure upon it from the injected material with subsequent vascular occlusion and infarction. Promotion of wound healing with semi-occlusive dressings and antibiotics is the only treatment. Transient erythema, swelling and bruising may occur occasionally.

Fibrel

The product consists of a small amount of the patient's plasma added to highly purified denatured porcine collagen (gelatin) and ε-aminocaproic acid to prevent digestion by fibrinolysin of fibrin deposits upon the gelatin matrix.[35] The injection of Fibrel is comparable to that used for injectable bovine collagen. Superficial placement of the material increases longevity and overcorrection of about 50 per cent is encouraged. Local anaesthesia or regional nerve blocks are required prior to injection to reduce the discomfort, which is greater than that accompanying Zyderm/Zyplast or silicone. The mode of

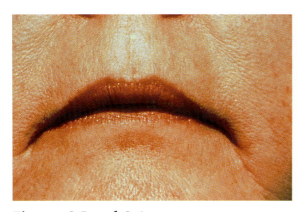 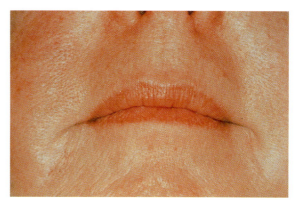

Figures 8.5 and 8.6
Before and after pictures of softform implants, lips (expanded polytetrafluoroethylene – EPTFE) (courtesy of Collagen corporation).

action of Fibrel is presumed to involve fibroblast activation with subsequent collagen deposition.

Side-effects[35] include an immediate urticarial reaction with erythema and swelling at the treatment sites, usually subsiding in 24–48 hours. Punctate bruising for a few days may also occur. Skin testing should be performed in all patients at least 1 month prior to treatment, but allergic reactions are rare since the gelatin is highly denatured and minimally antigenic.

All these techniques may be helpful for the treatment of facial lines and wrinkles provided the patients are selected carefully, thoroughly counselled and well informed of the limitations of this therapeutic approach.[29]

Others

Some of them have given encouraging clinical results for augmentation of rhytids, nasolabial folds and lips. Hyaluronic acid is used for the treatment of wrinkles (Figures 8.1 and 8.2). Alloderm provides a supple and natural feeling tissue filler. Expanded polytetrafluoroethylene (EPTFE) also serves as a supple tissue filler and can be removed completely if an adverse reaction develops (Figures 8.3–8.6).

Microliposuction and autologous fat transplantation

Removal of fat by microliposuction from areas where it has accumulated can enhance and rejuvenate the aging face. Similarly fat replacement through autologous fat transplantation can also rejuvenate the aging face, giving it a less angular, more rounded appearance.[37]

Microlipoinjection is autologous fat transplantation. Briefly, the fat should be removed from areas that usually respond the least to diet or exercise, such as the trochanteric areas, upper medial thighs, hips and periumbilical area.[38] It should be aspirated from the deeper layer of fat, which is genetically and metabolically different from the more superficial one.[39] After local anaesthesia, the fat is

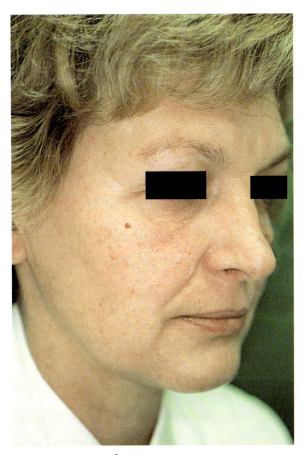 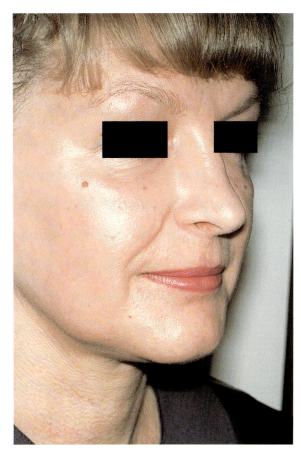

Figures 8.7 and 8.8
Before and pictures of Baker's phenol peel (courtesy of Dr Alastair Carruthers).

extracted with a syringe using either a needle or a microlipoextractor, or microcannula. After extraction, the syringe is placed in a centrifuge and rotated for 2–3 seconds to separate the excess fluid (blood and local anaesthetic) from the triglycerides released by broken adipocytes and from the fat ready to be transplanted.[37] After anaesthesia of the recipient area, the needle is inserted into the subcutaneous layer of the area to be corrected, and the fat injected until the defect is completely corrected. This procedure may be useful to correct defects of the glabellar area of the nasolabial grooves and commissures of the upper and lower lips, and the malar and submalar areas and cheeks.

Extraction of the fat may be associated with subcutaneous haemorrhage and irregularities at the donor site, as well as injuries to vital structures and infection. Several sessions are required for a maintenance of correction. Fifty to seventy per cent of the first autologous fat transplant is absorbed within 3–4 weeks. Then a second session is required to fill the defect as well as a third session 3–6 months later. Further transplantation may be needed

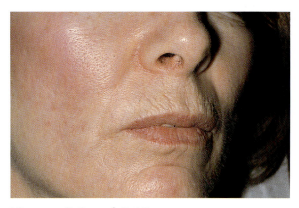 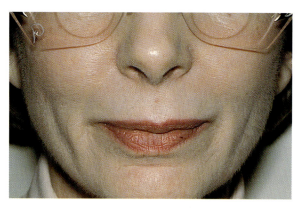

Figures 8.9 and 8.10

Before and pictures of laser resurfacing (courtesy of Dr Alastair Carruthers).

for up to 2 years after the initial transplantation.[37]

Because liposuction of the face is performed with small-diameter instruments and little fat may be removed, it may be termed microliposuction.[38] Local anaesthesia with adequate haemostasis is required, with oral sedation or analgesia or intravenous sedation by an anesthetist. This technique may be applied to various areas of the face, including the neck, specifically the undersurface of the maxilla and the anterosuperior aspect of the neck, the jowls, the cheeks and the malar pouches. This technique has a great potential for significant damage to the vasculature and the nerves present in the area of facial liposuction. Side-effects include unsightly indentation or irregularities due to excessive liposuction, deep haemorrhage, nerve damage, postinflammatory hyperpigmentation or localized haemosiderosis. This technique should be attempted only by well-trained and experienced surgeons.

Chemical peeling

The main indication for chemical facial peeling is treatment of sundamaged skin. Different peeling agents cause destruction to various depths of the epidermis. As discussed previously (concerning α-hydroxy acids), high concentrations of α-hydroxy acids (50–75%) have clinical utility as peeling agents. Resorcin produces a predictable and reproducible mild exfoliation. Jessner's solution (Resorcinol 14 g, salicylic acid 14 g, lactic acid 14 c^2, QS ethanol 100 c^2) can also be used to produce a superficial peel. Trichloroacetic acid (TCA) can result in variable wounding depth. A 15–25% solution of TCA will produce superficial destruction of epidermis. When used in a 45% solution, TCA produces epidermal necrosis and partial dermal denaturation. The phenol peel is a very effective method for improving actinically damaged skin due to the great depth of exfoliation (Figures 8.7 and 8.8). The Baker–Gordon formula, which contains approximately 48% phenol, is the most commonly used.

Superficial chemical peels do not play a major role in the treatment of the aging face. They are very useful for skin revitalization, with their greatest contribution being improvement of skin mottling and fine facial lines. Medium-depth and deep peels, either as sole procedures or in combination with other facial surgery, can produce a dramatic

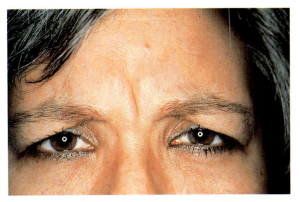

Figure 8.11

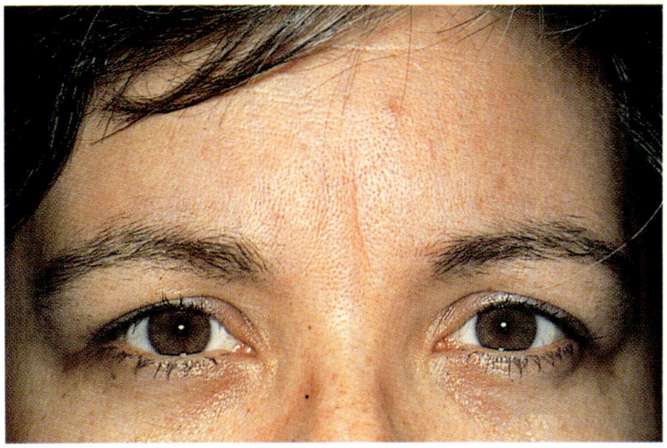

Figure 8.12

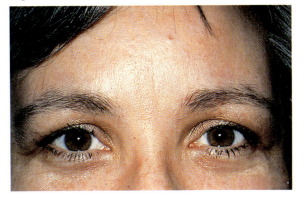

Figure 8.13

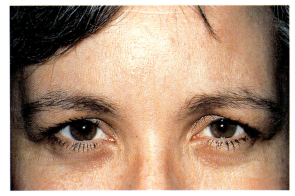

Figure 8.14

Figures 8.11, 8.12, 8.13, 8.14
Before and after pictures (at rest and growing) of Botulinum toxin to the glabellar folds (courtesy of Dr Alastair Carruthers).

improvement in solar elastosis, rhytides and selected pigmentary anomalies.

A recent controlled study compared the efficacy of a medium-depth chemical peel using 40% TCA with and without tretinoin, taking data from before (6 weeks) and after (4–5 months) treatment.[39] Overall, 40% TCA, even with tretinoin, does not dramatically reverse the manifestations of photodamage in most patients, although some improvement was noted in all patients. There was moderate and occasionally marked improvement with respect to lentigines, actinic keratoses, texture and overall appearance. Wrinkles were least affected. No statistically significant difference was found between patients treated with TCA and tretinoin and those with TCA alone.

After a medium-depth chemical peel of photodamaged skin, ultrastructural examination reveals profound changes. The number of elastic fibres is reduced and numerous mature activated fibroblasts with prominent cytoplasm and organelles are present in the region of abundant new collagen deposition. These morphological observations suggest that an

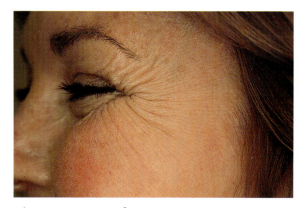 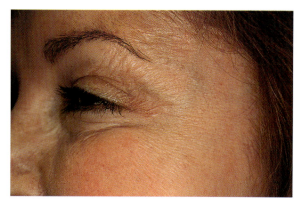

Figures 8.15 and 8.16
Before and pictures of Botulinum toxin to the Crow's feet (courtesy of Dr Alastair Carruthers).

increased synthesis of dermal matrix macromolecules occurs following peeling. This has been confirmed by sodium dodecyl sulphate gel electrophoresis of pepsin-digested skin biopsy showing a marked increased of collagen type I.[40]

Dermabrasion

Patients with moderate to severe photodamage can be treated with a mid-to-deep dermal surgical planing of the face. Dermabrasion consists of application of diamond fraises or motor-driven steel wire brushes to the skin with a deliberate attempt to wound the epidermis and the papillary dermis. In addition to the beneficial therapeutic value for aged and photodamaged skin, dermabrasion has recently been demonstrated to be a valid means of prophylaxis against neoplastic changes.[41] In patients with significant photoaging treated with full-face dermabrasion, histological examination demonstrates that this procedure can eliminate for many years the observed abnormal epidermal and dermal changes of photodamaged skin. After treatment, a revitalized papillary dermal Grenz zone of new collagen and new elastic tissue is observed and may account for the clinical improvement. Immunohistological examination demonstrates a dramatic increase of papillary dermal fibroblast staining for procollagen I a few weeks post-dermabrasion.[42] Western blotting demonstrated an increase in procollagen I that was corroborated by in situ hybridization. These observations suggest that the ability of dermabrasion clinically to improve photoaged skin may in large part be due to increased collagen I synthesis.[42]

Manual resurfacing combined with 25% trichloroacetic acid is also used to treat patients with extensive photodamage and widespread actinic keratoses. Manual resurfacing is performed by moving sandpaper or cautery tip cleaner, which has been moistened with sterile saline and wrapped around a gauze, against the skin. This technique produces excellent cosmetic results. Histologically, treated skin shows replacement of the dermal elastotic band by newly formed collagen.[43]

Laser skin resurfacing

Carbon dioxide (CO_2) laser skin resurfacing has been used by the practising dermatologist for over a decade[44] for the treatment of facial actinic damage. However, resurfacing with conventional continuous-wave CO_2 laser at low fluence gives a very narrow therapeutic range with predictable complications due to significant thermal injury to the dermis and adnexal structures, leading to permanent or long-term changes such as scarring and pigment changes.

The recent development of high-peak-power short-exposure-time CO_2 lasers allows for the delivery of char-free ablation, for a more controlled and therefore safer means of tissue resurfacing. The ultrapulse CO_2 laser can deliver energy of up to 500 mJ per pulse and has the ability to be pulsed at an interval shorter than the thermal relaxation time of the skin (695–950 ms). A computerized scanning device, the computerized pattern generator, may be combined with the ultrapulse CO_2 laser. This procedure provides more rapid resurfacing (15 minutes for full-face resurfacing compared with approximately 1 hour for freehand delivery). Furthermore, pulses are delivered with more uniformity leading to more rapid resurfacing. The Silk Touch Flashscanner, a CO_2 laser accessory, uses software-driven technology to create char-free ablation by sharply focusing the beam for a high-power density and rapidly moving the beam in a spiral pattern for a short exposure time. The scan takes place at a rapid rate (0.2 seconds for one cycle) to prevent the time spent positioned at any one particular point from being more than the thermal relaxation time of the skin. The anesthesia used consists of a variety of techniques such as EMLA cream, effective for two and sometimes up to three passes, and regional blocks or local infiltration with lidocaine for deeper ablations or more sensitive patients. General anaesthesia or intravenous sedation may be required for full-face ablations.

Laser skin resurfacing has become a very promising treatment for actinically damaged skin. Both the ultrapulse CO_2 laser and the Silk Touch Flashscanner are effective for skin resurfacing of photodamaged facial skin.[45,46] In 100 patients with different severities of photodamaged skin undergoing treatment with the ultrapulse CO_2 laser, 68 showed a moderate improvement and 5 a marked improvement at 1 month post-laser treatment. By 2 months post-laser treatment, 20 of the remaining 27 patients achieved a moderate to marked improvement from baseline.[45] Significant improvement of facial rhytides was observed in 40 patients treated using the Silk Touch Flashscanner attached to one of the two continuous-wave CO_2 lasers (Sharplan 1030 or Surgipulse XJ 150). Optical micrometry evaluation of silicone replicas obtained pre- and 2 months post-laser treatment confirmed the clinical observations.[46]

Facial rhytides, both perioral and periorbital wrinkles, respond well to laser resurfacing with 50 per cent improvement (Figures 8.9 and 8.10).[47] Nasolabial folds respond poorly. Patients tend to do better when entire anatomical units are treated, such as the entire perioral area or the entire periorbital area. Patients usually heal in approximately 7–10 days. The most frequent complications are persistent erythema and postinflammatory hyperpigmentation. Postoperative erythema usually averages 6 weeks, but can last several months. The duration of this side-effect has direct correlation with the depth of ablation.[45] Postinflammatory hyperpigmentation correlates with the skin type of the patient and is rarely seen in skin types I and II. However, laser skin resurfacing can be performed on darker skin types with caution and proper pre- or postoperative treatments.[47] In patients where hyperpigmentation is a concern, topical bleaching agents containing retinoic acid and/or α-hydroxy acids are started 2 weeks prior to the procedure. These agents are restarted a few days to a couple of weeks after complete healing. However, caution must be exercised in restarting these agents in case of irritation. Patients are instructed to avoid sun exposure after the procedure and are placed on a sunscreen. In 30 Asian or Hispanic patients (skin types III and IV) treated by laser resurfacing, hyperpigmentation occurred but was reduced by regular use of tretinoin, hydroquinone and desonide cream both pre- and postoperatively, along with use of broad-spectrum sunscreens after treatments.[47] Hypopigmentation does not occur in patients treated with one to three passes. This side-effect is attributed to deeper follicular melanocyte injury, which should not occur with laser resurfacing. Great care is needed to avoid contact irritancy with topical agents, which not only results in discomfort and longer recovery times but also increases the chance of postoperative erythema and hyperpigmentation. Pretreatment of all patients with the minimal amount of topical therapy should be recommended. Moisturizers must be selected to have the fewest preservatives and the lowest risk of irritancy. Prevention of cutaneous infections should be carried out using broad-spectrum antibiotics and oral antiherpes therapy.[45]

Histological evaluation of treated sites shows removal of the epidermis with minimal residual thermal necrosis after the initial pass and penetration into the papillary dermis after the second pass. Further passes show full-thickness ablation of the papillary dermis (third) or ablation of the reticular dermis (fourth).[46] The mechanisms of CO_2 laser resurfacing are regeneration of dermis and epidermis as well as collagen remodelling. Improvement attained even with relatively superficial ablation suggests that collagen shrinkage due to a thermal effect may be involved in the skin improvement.[45]

Laser skin resurfacing is still a relatively new technique and further refinements are needed. Available data suggest that this technique permits better control and reproducibility in cutaneous resurfacing than previously available chemical peels and dermabrasion.[47] The procedure is much cleaner and neater, and does not carry the same risk as previously available techniques.

Aesthetic surgery

A large variety of effective surgical procedures for achieving facial rejuvenation is currently available. Loss of adherence of the skin to subcutaneous tissues together with gravity effects and fat redistribution in the periorbital region, mandibular line and anterior cervical area contributes to the sagging appearance of the face.[48]

Rejuvenation surgery of the areas requires not only repositioning and excision of the excess skin, but also removal of the excess and abnormal fat deposits.[48] It is beyond the objectives of this monograph to describe the surgical guidelines of these procedures.

Facelift or rhytidectomy rejuvenates primarily the lower third of the face and upper neck. Complications of facelift surgery include haematoma (occurring in 4–15% of the patients), skin slough, generalized face and neck ecchymosis, facial nerve injuries, pain, alopecia in the temporal and postauricular areas and hypertrophic scarring.[49] Because rhytidectomy does not affect the eyes and the upper third of the face, it often accompanies blepharoplasty or forehead lift. Upper lid and lower lid blepharoplasty may be performed. Complications include temporary or permanent ectropion, blindness, ptosis and lagophthalmus.

For the upper part of the face, several types of forehead lift may be performed, the coronal lift, the temporal lift or the mid-forehead lift, depending on the changes.[50] Complications of these procedures include haematoma formation, alopecia, sensory changes and lagophtalmus.

Botulinum toxin (BT)

BT is a neurotoxin that prevents the release of acetylcholine at the neuromuscular junction and produces reversible paralysis of striated muscle. BT was initially used in human beings as therapy for strabismus. The first use of BT for cosmetic indications was reported in the early 1990s. The idea of using BT for the correction of wrinkle lines arose from the observation that BT therapy for facial dystonias markedly decreased lines and wrinkles in the treated areas.[51,52]

BT is mainly used for the treatment of glabellar wrinkles (Figures 8.11–8.14). Vertical glabellar frown lines are the result of overactivity of the corrugator superciliaris muscles with contribution from both the procerus and orbicularis oculi muscles. The only function of this muscle is to draw the eyebrows inferomedially as an expression of emotion. Paralysis of the central brow musculature eliminates this. In addition, unopposed action of the medial elevators of the brow produces a 'medial brow lift'. The glabellar furrows are treated with intramuscular injection of 25 U of BT following a five-step process in women. Men require seven injections and 35 U. Some investigators recommend the use of electromyographic guidance to allow an accurate localization of functioning muscles. Successful therapy is signalled by muscle weakening that begins 24–48 hours after the session, peaking at up to 7 days. Once the forehead is smooth, the patient is instructed to return for therapy when he or she notices a return of muscle movement, which may not occur for 4 months to 1 year or even longer.

BT treatment is also used for crow's-feet (Figures 8.15 and 8.16), horizontal forehead lines, mesolabial folds and other hyperkinetic facial lines. These lines are the result of physiologically important facial muscle weakeners and complete paralysis is not the end-point sought. For these purposes, BT is injected subcutaneously rather than intramuscularly and the amount injected is smaller (i.e. 1–2 U per site).

This form of therapy is remarkably safe. Allergic or urticarial lesions have not been reported. Transient bruising at the injection site or brief pain or headache following injection may occur. Transient ptosis probably resulting from local dissemination of toxin at the injection site is the most significant complication of injection in the glabellar area. If guidelines to avoid this side-effect are carefully followed, ptosis, if it occurs at all, will be minimal and short-lived.

BT should not be injected in either pregnant or lactating women. Other contraindications include a previous history of a neuromuscular condition and concomitant use of aminoglycosides, which potentiate the effects of BT therapy.

The therapy is effective for facial wrinkles caused by hyperkinetic muscles of expression and satisfies both physician and patients. BT as botulinum type A purified neurotoxin is approved in the US for the treatment of some neurological and ophthalmological conditions, but its use for cosmetic application is not approved.

Prevention

Sunscreens and photoprotection

Experimental studies in animals have demonstrated that some sunscreens are capable of providing protection against ultraviolet-induced photoaging. Sunscreens produce striking and dose-dependent reduction in photoaging-like dermal damage and reduce photocarcinogenesis in the ultraviolet-irradiated hairless mouse model. Application of sun protection factor (SPF) 15 sunscreen completely prevents heliodermatitis in hairless mice irradiated with sunlamps emitting UVA and UVB simultaneously.[53] Substantial repair of the elastosis resulting from 20 weeks of UVB irradiation occurs during a subsequent 10 weeks of UVB irradiation if the animals are protected during the second irradiation period by an SPF-15 sunscreen[54] In hairless mice irradiated with UVA and UVA/UVB after application of sunscreens, UVB induces the most histological changes, such as epidermal thickening, dermal inflammation and elastic fibre changes.[55] Applications of UVB sunscreens alone significantly reduce these changes and the addition of a UVA sunscreen further diminishes epidermal thickening, elastic fibre loss/hyperplasia and dermal inflammation.[55]

Only one study reports the effects of long-term use of a topical UVA/UVB sunscreen to prevent the histological changes of photodamage in humans.[56] Forty-six patients were given either sunscreen containing 7% octylethoxycinnamate (UVB blocker), 6% oxybenzone (UVA/350 nm blocker) and 5% octylsalicylate (UVB blocker) or vehicle to apply daily for 24 months. Punch biopsies obtained from preauricular skin at 12 and 24 months were examined by light microscopy and computer-generated analysis. The results demonstrate that the application of a sunscreen which blocks out UVB and shortwave UVA significantly diminishes the progressive worsening of solar elastosis. In contrast to the case in irradiated hairless mice, no repair of solar elastosis was seen. Furthermore, no differences between the sunscreen and the placebo groups were noted with respect to dermal inflammation, epidermal thickening and keratinocyte atypia. Thus, the long-term use of a topical short-wave UVA/UVB sunscreen contributes significantly to the prevention of solar elastosis compared with placebo. Further studies using broad-spectrum sunscreens blocking UVB and the whole UVA range are urgently needed.

Two studies have demonstrated that the long-term use of UVA/UVB sunscreens induces a significant reduction in actinic keratoses.[57,58] From these data, it is likely that the routine use of effective sunscreens absorbing both UVA and UVB irradiation should be recommended to reduce both ultraviolet-induced skin carcinogenesis and photoaging in humans.[59] The cost of sunscreens may explain why they are not more often used. However, even when sunscreens are provided free of charge, only 35 per cent of people actually use them.[60] Several factors, including lack of knowledge about skin cancer and the other deleterious effects of sunlight on skin, and the culture of tanning, may be significant for this failure to employ sun protection.

Antioxidants

Chronic exposure of skin to UV radiation can significantly decrease cellular and membrane antioxidants,[61] and their depletion could lead to imperfect protection against cumulative stress of free radicals produced by chronic sun irradiation. A growing body of evidence suggests that reactive oxygen species are generated by ultraviolet irradiation, resulting in structural and functional alterations of cutaneous components which should affect the photoaging process over a long period.[62] Therefore, supplementation of skin with antioxidants should prevent radical-mediated oxidative skin damage and perhaps reduce or prevent photodamage. Several antioxidants have been readily proved to work under experimental conditions and in laboratory animals.

Non-enzymatic antioxidants include the lipid-soluble molecules tocopherol (vitamin E); β-carotene, a precursor of vitamin A; and ascorbic acid. α-Tocopherol, the most active form of vitamin E, breaks free radical chain reactions and inhibits already initiated peroxidation. In an animal model, topically applied tocopherol is protective against skin photoaging.[63]

Ascorbic acid (vitamin C) is the main water-soluble non-enzymatic antioxidant. It interacts with a wide variety of free radicals intracellularly and is an ideal free radical scavenger. In addition, ascorbate plays an important role in the regeneration of α-tocopherol from the tocopherol radical in skin. Thus, ascorbic acid not only directly protects membranes and low-density lipoproteins from reactive oxygen species generated in the aqueous phase, but also indirectly protects them by reduction of the vitamin E radical. Vitamin C has the additional advantage of stimulating dermal fibroblasts to synthesize collagen, a major target of photoaging. Animal studies have shown significant acute photoprotective and chronic photoaging preventive effects from topical application. Despite this information, no clinical trials have been carried out to evaluate the potential of topical vitamin C in the prevention and treatment of photoaging.

Topical application of certain iron chelators dramatically delays the onset of UVB radiation-induced skin photodamage in chronically UV-irradiated hairless mice.[64] These observations suggest that topical antioxidants could be of some help in the prevention of cutaneous photodamage. However, in placebo-controlled studies, oral vitamin E[65,66] or β-carotene supplementation do not decrease the severity of acute cutaneous photodamage in normal subjects.

Oestrogen

In post-menopausal women, oestrogen deficiency may contribute to the development of age-related changes such as skin atrophy, wrinkling, dryness, laxity and decreased collagen content. Several studies have suggested that oestrogen preserves skin collagen content, elastic properties and thickness. Results from a large population-based study strongly suggest that oestrogen use protects against some aspects of cutaneous aging. Among 3403 women receiving post-menopausal oestrogen therapy, a statistically significant decrease in the likelihood of senile dry skin was observed.[67] Furthermore the prevalence of wrinkling was lower in oestrogen users. These findings suggest that post-menopausal oestrogen therapy protects against skin wrinkling and dryness.

References

1. Kligman AM, Grove GL, Hirose R, Leyden JJ, Topical tretinoin for photoaged skin. *J Am Acad Dermatol* (1986) **15**: 838–59.
2. Weiss JS, Ellis CN, Headington JT et al, Topical tretinoin improves photoaged skin. *JAMA* (1988) **259**: 527–32.
3. Zelickson AS, Mottz, JH, Weiss JS et al, Topical tretinoin in photoaging: an ultrastructural study. *J Cut Aging Cosm Dermatol* (1988) **1**: 41–7.
4. Lever L, Kumar P, Marks R, Topical retinoic acid for treatment of solar damage. *Br J Dermatol* (1990) **122**: 91–8.
5. Leyden JJ, Grove GL, Grove MJ et al, Treatment of photodamaged facial skin with topical tretinoin. *J Am Acad Dermatol* (1989) **21**: 638–44.
6. Grove GL, Grove MJ, Leyden JJ et al, Skin replica analysis of photodamaged skin after therapy with tretinoin emollient cream. *J Am Acad Dermatol* (1991) **25**: 231–7.
7. Weinstein GD, Nigra TP, Pochi PE et al, Topical tretinoin for treatment of photodamaged skin. A multicenter study. *Arch Dermatol* (1991) **127**: 659–65.
8. Olsen EA, Katz I, Levine N et al, Tretinoin emollient cream: a new therapy for photodamaged skin. *J Am Acad Dermatol* (1992) **26**: 215–24.
9. Green LJ, McCormick A, Weinstein GD, Photoaging and the skin. The effects of tretinoin. *Dermatol Clin* (1993) **11**: 97–105.
10. Bhawan J, Olsen E, Lufrano L et al, Histologic evaluation of the long-term effects of tretinoin on photodamaged skin. *J Dermatol Sci* (1995) **11**: 177–82.
11. Kligman AM, Dogadkina D, Lavker RM, Effects of topical tretinoin on non-sun-exposed protected skin of the elderly. *J Am Acad Dermatol* (1993) **39**: 25–33.
12. Kligman AM, Guidelines for the use of topical tretinoin (Retin-A) for photoaged skin. *J Am Acad Dermatol* (1989) **21**: 650–4.
13. Griffiths CEM, Kang S, Ellis CN et al, Two concentrations of topical tretinoin (retinoic acid) cause similar improvement of photoaging but different degrees of irritation. *Arch Dermatol* (1995) **131**: 1037–44.
14. Duell EA, Anström A, Griffiths CE et al, Human skin levels of retinoic acid and cytochrome P450 derived 4-hydroxyretinoic

acid after topical application of retinoic acid in vivo compared to concentrations required to stimulate retinoic acid receptor-mediated transcription in vitro. *J Clin Invest* (1992) **90**: 1269–74.
15. Rees J, The molecular biology of retinoic acid receptors: orphan from good family seeks home. *Br J Dermatol* (1992) **126**: 97–104.
16. Fisher GJ, Esmann J, Griffiths CEM et al, Cellular immunologic and biochemical characterization of topical retinoic acid-treated human skin. *J Invest Dermatol* (1995) **61**: 223–47.
17. Elder JT, Fisher GJ, Zhang QY et al, Retinoic acid receptor gene expression in human skin. *J Invest Dermatol* (1991) **96**: 425–33.
18. Elder JT, Aström A, Petterson U et al, Retinoic acid receptors and binding proteins in human skin. *J Invest Dermatol* (1992) **98**: 36S–41S.
19. Fisher GJ, Talwar HS, Xiao JH et al, Immunological identification and functional quantitation of retinoic acid and retinoid X receptor proteins in human skin. *J Biol Chem* (1994) **269**: 20629–35.
20. Zhang LX, Mills KJ, Dawson MI et al, Evidence for the involvement of retinoic acid receptor RARα-dependent signalling pathway in the induction of tissue transglutaminase and apoptosis by retinoids. *J Biol Chem* (1995) **270**: 6022–9.
21. Xiao JH, Durand B, Chambon P, Voorhees JJ, Endogenous retinoic acid receptor (RAR)-retinoid X receptor (RXR) heterodimers are the major functional forms regulating retinoid-responsive elements in adult human keratinocytes. *J Biol Chem* (1995) **270**: 3001–11.
22. Sendagorta E, Lesiewicz J, Armstrong RB, Topical isotretinoin for photodamaged skin. *J Am Acad Dermatol* (1992) **27**: S15–S18.
23. Saurat JH, Didierjean L, Masgrau E et al, Topical retinaldehyde on human skin: biologic effects and tolerance. *J Invest Dermatol* (1994) **103**: 770–4.
24. Van Scott EJ, Ditre CM, Yu RJ, Alpha hydroxyacids in the treatment of signs of photoaging. *Clin Dermatol* (1996) **14**: 217–26.
25. Newman N, Newman A, Moy LS et al, Clinical improvement of photoaged skin with 50% glycolic acid. A double-blind vehicle-controlled study. *Dermatol Surg* (1996) **22**: 455–60.
26. Piacquadio D, Dobry M, Hunt S et al, Short contact 70% glycolic acid peels as a treatment for photodamaged skin. A pilot study. *Dermatol Surg* (1996) **22**: 449–42.
27. Ditre CM, Griffin TD, Murphy GF et al, Effects of α-hydroxy acids on photoaged skin: pilot clinical, histologic and ultrastructural study. *J Am Acad Dermatol* (1996) **34**: 187–95.
28. Smith WP, Epidermal and dermal effects of topical lactic acid. *J Am Acad Dermatol* (1996) **35**: 388–91.
29. Griffin TD, Murphy GF, Sueki H et al, Increased factor XIIIa transglutaminase expression in dermal dendrocytes after treatment with α-hydroxy acids: potential physiologic significance. *J Am Acad Dermatol* (1996) **34**: 196–203.
30. Pollack SV, Silicone, Fibrel and collagen implantation for facial lines and wrinkles. *J Dermatol Surg Oncol* (1990) **16**: 956–61.
31. Orentreich DS, Orentreich N, Injectable fluid silicone. In: Roenigk RK, Roenigk HH Jr (eds) *Dermatologic Surgery Principles and Practice.* Marcel Dekker: New York, 1989, pp. 1349–95.
32. Winer LH, Sternberg TH, Lehman R, Ashley FL, Tissue reaction to injected silicone liquids, a report of three cases. *Arch Dermatol* (1964) **90**: 588–93.
33. Stegman SJ, Chu S, Armstrong RC, Adverse reactions to bovine collagen implant: clinical and histologic features. *J Dermatol Surg Oncol* (1988) **14**: 39–48.
34. Stegman SJ, Chu S, Bensch K, Armstrong R, A light and electron microscopic evaluation of Zyderm collagen and Zyplast implants in aging human facial skin. *Arch Dermatol* (1987) **123**: 1644–9.
35. Spangler AS, Treatment of depressed cutaneous scars with fibrin foam – seventeen years of experience. *J Dermatol Surg Oncol* (1975) **1**: 65–9.
36. Millikan L, Long-term safety and efficacy with Fibrel in the treatment of cutaneous scars: results of a multicenter study. *J Dermatol Surg Oncol* (1989) **15**: 837–42.
37. Asken S, Microliposuction and autologous fat transplantation for aesthetic enhancement of the aging face. *J Dermatol Surg Oncol* (1990) **16**: 965–72.
38. Asken SF, Facial liposuction and microlipoinjection. *J Dermatol Surg Oncol* (1988) **14**: 297–305.

39. Humphreys TR, Werth V, Dzubow L, Kligman A, Treatment of photodamaged skin with trichloroacetic acid and topical tretinoin. *J Am Acad Dermatol* (1996) **34**: 638–44.
40. Nelson BR, Fader DJ, Gillard M et al, Pilot histologic and ultrastructural study of the effects of medium-depth chemical facial peels on dermal collagen in patients with actinically damaged skin. *J Am Acad Dermatol* (1995) **32**: 472–8.
41. Benedetto AV, Griffin TD, Benedetto EA et al, Dermabrasion: therapy and prophylaxis of the photoaged skin. *J Am Acad Dermatol* (1992) **27**: 439–47.
42. Nelson BR, Griffiths CE, Gillard MO et al, Clinical improvement following dermabrasion of photoaged skin correlates with synthesis of collagen. I. *Arch Dermatol* (1994) **130**: 1136–42.
43. Cooley JE, Casey DL, Kauffman CL, Manual resurfacing and trichloroacetic acid for the treatment to patients with widespread actinic damage. *Dermatol Surg* (1997) **23**: 373–9.
44. David LM, Sarne AJ, Unger WP, Rapid laser scanning for facial resurfacing. *Dermatol Surg* (1995) **21**: 1031–3.
45. Lowe NJ, Lask G, Griffin ME et al, Skin resurfacing with the ultrapulse carbon dioxide laser. Observations on 100 patients. *Dermatol Surg* (1995) **21**: 1025–9.
46. Lask G, Keller G, Lowe N, Gormley D, Laser skin resurfacing with the silk Touch flashscanner for facial rhytides. *Dermatol Surg* (1995) **21**: 1021–4.
47. Ho C, Nguyen Q, Lowe NJ et al, Laser resurfacing in pigmented skin. *Dermatol Surg* (1995) **21**: 1035–7.
48. David L, Lask G, Laser cosmetic surgery. *Dermatol Surg* (1995) **21**: 1015.
49. Fuleihan NS, Webster RC, Smith RC, The face lift and ancillary procedures. *J Dermatol Surg Oncol* (1990) **16**: 975–87.
50. Tardy ME Jr, Parras G, Schwartz M, Aesthetic surgery of the face. *Dermatol Clin* (1991) **9**: 169–87.
51. Klein AW, Cosmetic therapy with botulinum toxin. Anecdotal memoirs. *Dermatol Surg* (1996) **22**: 757–9.
52. Carruthers A, Kiene K, Carruthers J, Botulinum: an exotoxin use in clinical dermatology. *J Am Acad Dermatol* (1996) **34**: 788–97.
53. Kligman LH, Akin FJ, Kligman AM, Prevention of ultraviolet damage to the dermis of hairless mice by sunscreens. *J Invest Dermatol* (1982) **78**: 181–9.
54. Kligman LH, Akin FJ, Kligman AM, Sunscreens promote repair of ultraviolet radiation-induced dermal damage. *J Invest Dermatol* (1983) **81**: 98–102.
55. Harrison JA, Walfer SL, Plastow R, Sunscreens with low sun protection factor inhibit ultraviolet B and A photoaging in the skin of the hairless albino mouse. *Photoderm Photoimmunol Photomed* (1991) **8**: 12–20.
56. Boyd AS, Nayloe M, Cameron GS et al, The effects of chronic sunscreen use on the histologic changes of dermatoheliosis. *J Am Acad Dermatol* (1995) **33**: 941–6.
57. Naylor MF, Boyd A, Smith DW et al, High sun protection factor sunscreens in the suppression of actinic neoplasia. *Arch Dermatol* (1995) **131**: 170–5.
58. Thompson SC, Jolley D, Marks R, Reduction of solar keratoses by regular sunscreen use. *N Engl J Med* (1993) **329**: 1147–51.
59. Lowe NJ, Sunscreens and the prevention of skin aging. *J Dermatol Surg Oncol* (1990) **16**: 936–8.
60. Johnson EY, Lookingbill DP, Sunscreen use and sun exposure: trends in a white population. *Arch Dermatol* (1984) **120**: 727–31.
61. Maeda K, Naganuma M, Fukusa M, Effects of chronic exposure ultraviolet-A including 2% ultraviolet-B on free radical reduction systems in hairless mice. *Photochem Photobiol* (1991) **54**: 737–40.
62. Miyachi Y, Photoaging from an oxidative standpoint. *J Dermatol Sci* (1995) **9**: 79–86.
63. Jurkiewicz BA, Bissett DL, Buettner GR, Effect of topically applied tocopherol on ultraviolet radiation-mediated free radical damage in skin. *J Invest Dermatol* (1995) **104**: 484–8.
64. Bissett DL, Chaterjee R, Hannon DP, Chronic ultraviolet radiation increase in skin, iron and the photoprotective effect of topically iron chelators. *Photochem Photobiol* (1991) **54**: 215–23.
65. Garmyn M, Ribaya-Mercado JD, Russel RM et al, Effect of beta-carotene supplementation on the human sunburn reaction. *Exp Dermatol* (1995) **4**: 104–11.
66. Werninghaus K, Meydani M, Bhawan J et al,

Evaluation of the photoprotective effect of oral vitamin E supplementation. *Arch Dermatol* (1994) **130**: 1257–61.

67. Dunn LB, Damesyn M, Moore AA et al, Does estrogen prevent skin aging? *Arch Dermatol* (1997) **133**: 339–42.

Index

Acantholytic solar keratosis, 68, 69
N-Acetyl-cysteine, 105-6
Acral lentiginous melanoma, 41
Actinic dermatitis, chronic, 102-3
Actinic granuloma, 16
Actinic keratoses, see Solar keratoses
Actinic lentigo (solar/senile lentigo), 31-3
   treatment, 57, 58, 112
      measuring effects, 112
Actinic porokeratosis, disseminated superficial, 71
Actinic prurigo, 100
Aesthetic surgery, 136
Aging (intrinsic/chronological), 20-1, 83-96
   dopa-positive melanocytes and, 46, 88
   dyspigmentation disorders, 46-7
      idiopathic guttate hypomelanosis, 45
   photoaging compared with, 93-4
   tretinoin use, 123
Aging (sun-induced), see Photoaging
Allergy, photo-, 104
All-*trans* retinoic acid, see Tretinoin
Aloe barbadensis extract, 104
α-hydroxy acids, 126-7, 132
   clinical studies, 126-7
      photodysplasia, 79
      pigmented lesions, 56-7
   mechanism of action, 127
Ammonium lactate, 57
Antioxidants, 105, 138-9
Ascorbic acid (vitamin C), 105, 138-9
Autologous fat transplantation, 130-2

Baker–Gordon phenol peel, 132
Basal cell carcinoma/epithelioma (rodent ulcer), 76-8
   clinical types, 76-8
      pigmented, 35-6, 77
   pathology, 78
Basal cell naevus syndrome, 63
Bcl-2, 49-50
Blisters in solar elastosis, 16
Blood flow changes, 113-14

Blood vessels
   aging, 90
   solar elastosis, 23
Boston skin type classification, 11, 12
Botulinum toxin, 136-7
Bovine collagen implants, 128-9
Bowen's disease, 70-1
Bullous solar elastosis, 16

Calcitonin gene-related peptide and UV, 99
Cancer, see also Premalignant lesions
   melanoma, see Melanoma
   non-melanoma, 35-6, 74-9, see also specific
      histological types
      treatment, 79
   pathogenesis, see Carcinogenesis
Carbon dioxide laser skin resurfacing, 134-5
Carcinogenesis, UV role (photocarcinogenesis), 98-100
   melanocytes, 40, 50-1
   non-melanoma cancer, 60-4, 74, 75, 79
Carcinoma
   basal cell, see Basal cell carcinoma
   sebaceous gland, 78-9
   squamous cell, see Squamous cell carcinoma
   sweat gland, 78-9
   trabecular, 79
Carcinoma segregans, 68, 69
CFCs and ozone destruction, 2
Chlorofluorocarbons and ozone destruction, 2
Chromameter, 112
Citrine skin, 12-13, 112
Civatte's disease, 36-8
Clinical measurements, 116-18
Clothing, 7
Collagen, aging and, 89
Collagen implants, 128-9
Colour changes, see also Pigmentary change
   measuring, 112-13
   solar elastosis, 12-13
Comedones, senile, 17-18
Connective tissue in aging, 88-90
Corneocytes and aging, 86

Index

Cosmetics, 127
Crow's feet, 12, 116
  treatment, 137
Cryotherapy
  actinic lentigo, 56
  idiopathic guttate hypomelanosis, 45
  lentigo maligna, 40
Cultural factors, 7-8
Cutaneous extrinsic aging score, 20
Cutaneous horn, 66, 69
Cutis rhomboidalis nuchae, 15
Cutometer, *see* Suction devices
Cytokines, melanocyte effects, 50

Darier-like keratosis, 68, 69
Decorin, 89
Degenerative change, solar elastotic, *see* Solar elastosis
Delayed hypersensitivity and UV, 98, 99
Dendritic cells and aging, 88
Depigmenting agents, 57
Dermis
  elastosis, *see* Elastosis
  intrinsic aging, 88-90
    compared with photoaging, 93
  surgical planning (dermabrasion), 57, 134
Dermo-epidermal junction and aging, 90-1
Discoid lupus erythematosus, 104
  actinic keratosis and, differentiation, 66-7
Discoloration, *see* Colour changes
Disulphide (S-S) bonds and solar elastosis, 24
DNA
  aging and, 84
  damage, 62-3
Dopa-positive melanocytes and aging, 46, 88
Drug phototoxicity, 103-4
Drug therapy, 121-30, *see also specific drugs*
  chronic actinic dermatitis, 103
  photodysplasia, 79
  pigmentary change, 51-6
    lentigo maligna, 40
    measuring effects, 112
    senile lentigo, 57, 58, 112
  polymorphic light eruption, 101-2
Dubreuilh's melanosis, *see* Lentigo maligna
Dyspigmentation, *see* Pigmentary change
Dysplasia (photodysplasia), epidermal, 63-4, *see also* Minimal dysplastic change
  treatment, 79

Elastin, 25

Elastosis
  defined, 21
  in erythema ab igne, 6
  linear focal, 16
  measuring degree of, 114-15
  solar, *see* Solar elastosis
Elderly skin, mechanical alterations, 90, *see also* Aging *and entries under* Senile
Emollients, 127
Endothelin-1, 50
  seborrhoeic keratoses and, 48
Enzyme activities, epidermal, 110
Ephelides, *see* Freckle
Epidermis
  dermis and, aging and area between, 90-1
  dysplasia, *see* Dysplasia
  intrinsic aging, 84-8
    compared with photoaging, 93
  solar elastosis and, 25
Epithelioma
  basal cell, *see* Basal cell carcinoma
  intraepidermal, 70-1
  self-healing, *see* Ferguson Smith self-healing epithelioma; Keratoacanthoma
  squamous cell, *see* Squamous cell carcinoma
Erythema
  assessment, 113
  solar elastosis, 14-15
Erythema ab igne, 6, 21
Erythrosis interfollicularis colli, 36-8
Ethnic groups, UVR injury predisposition, 12
Experimental models
  chronic UVR exposure, 20
  hair depigmentation, 49
  solar elastosis, 25-6

Facial rejuvenation, 136
Fat removal and replacement, 130-2
Favre–Racouchot syndrome, 17-18
Ferguson Smith self-healing epithelioma, 73-4
Fibrel, 129-30
Fibroblasts and aging, 89
Fibroxanthoma, atypical, 79
Forehead lift, 136
Freckle (ephelides), 30-1
  Hutchinson's, *see* Lentigo maligna
Free radical damage, 84
Freezing, *see* Cryotherapy
Freudenthal's funnel, 65

Genetic factor, hair depigmentation, 49

Glabellar folds, botulinum toxin, 137
Glucose-6-phosphate dehydrogenase, 62, 110
Glycolic acid, 56-7, 126
Gorlin's (basal cell naevus syndrome), 63
Granuloma
  actinic, 16
  lepromin-induced, 100
Grenz zone, 22
Grey hair, *see* Hair
Guttate hypomelanosis, idiopathic, 42-5

Hair, greying and whitening, 48-50, 87
Hairless mouse, elastotic degenerative change, 26
Halmi's stain, 21, 24, 115
Heat-related erythema (e. ab igne), 6, 21
Heredity and hair depigmentation, 49
Hormone (oestrogen) replacement therapy, 139
Horn, cutaneous, 66, 69
Horny layer of epidermis (stratum corneum), age-related change, 86
Hutchinson's freckle, *see* Lentigo maligna
Hutchinson's summer prurigo, 100
Hyaluronic acid, 130
Hydroquinone, 57
α-Hydroxy acids, *see under* alpha
Hypermelanotic lesions, *see* Hyperpigmented and hypermelanotic lesions
Hyperpigmented and hypermelanotic lesions, 29-42
  seborrhoeic keratoses, 47-50
  treatment, *see* Treatment
Hypersensitivity, delayed, UV and, 98, 99
Hypomelanotic lesions, 42-6

Immune response, UV/solar-induced changes, 63, 97-107
Immunosuppression
  age-related, 92
  UV/solar-induced, 63, 98-100
Implants, 127-30
Inflammation and aging, 91-3
Inflammatory cells
  actinic keratosis, 65-6
  Bowen's disease, 71
  solar elastosis, 23, 25
Infrared radiation, 6
Injectable liquid silicone, 127-8
Injury to deeper tissue, aging skin and, 90, 91-2
'Ink-spot' lentigines, 32-3
Interleukin-10 and UV, 99

Interleukin-12 and UV, 99-100
Intraepidermal epithelioma, 70-1
Isotretinoin (13-*cis*-retinoic acid) use, 125
  photodysplasia, 9

Jessner's solution, 57, 132

Keratinocytes
  age effects, 85, 86
  UV effects, 50
Keratoacanthoma (molluscum sebaceum; self-healing epithelioma), 72-3
  pigmented, 36
Keratoses, *see also* Porokeratosis
  Darier-like, 68, 69
  hyperpigmented seborrhoeic, 47-50
  hypopigmented, disseminated, 44
  LE-like, 66, 69
  solar, *see* Solar keratoses
Kidney transplantation and skin cancer, 99

Lactic acid, 126, 127
Langerhans' cells
  aging and, 88
  UV and, 99
Laser Doppler flowmeter, 114
Laser skin resurfacing, *see* Resurfacing
Leisure activities, outdoor, 7
Lentiginous melanoma, acral, 41
Lentigo/lentigenes
  actinic, *see* Actinic lentigo
  'ink-spot', 32-3
  UVA, 33-4
Lentigo maligna (Dubreuilh's melanosis; Hutchinson's melanotic freckle), 39-41
Lentigo maligna melanoma (LMM), 39, 40
Lepromin-induced granulomas, 100
Lichenoid solar keratoses, 67, 69
Light mice, 49
Linear focal elastosis, 16
Lipoinjection, micro-, 130-2
Liposuction, micro-, 130-2
Lupus erythematosus, 104
  discoid, *see* Discoid lupus erythematosus
Lupus erythematosus-like keratosis, 66, 69
Lymphocytes and UV, 99, 100
Lymphomas and UV, 98
Lysozyme and solar elastosis, 25

Malignancy, *see* Cancer
Measuring photodamage, 109-19

Mechanical alterations
  aging skin, 90
  sun-damaged skin, 18-21, 116
Melanin
  in seborrhoeic keratoses, 48
  synthesis, retinoic acid and, 52-3
Melanin Meter (Mexameter), 112, 113
Melanocytes (pigment cells in skin)
  dopa-positive, aging and, 46, 88
  grey hair and, 48-9
  melanogenesis in, retinoic acid and, 52-3
  UVR effects, 50-1
Melanocytic naevi, 38-9
  age-related changes in number, 46-7
Melanoma, 41-2
  holidays and, 8
  lentigo maligna (LMM), 39, 40
  UV role in pathogenesis, 40, 50-1
Melanoma cell lines, retinoic acid effects, 52-6
Merkel cell tumour, 79
Metastases, squamous cell carcinoma, 74-5
Mexameter, 112, 113
Mice, see Mouse
Microlipoinjection, 130-2
Microliposuction, 130-2
Microsatellite instability, 62-3
Minimal dysplastic change, 64
  prevalence/significance, 68-9
Models, see Experimental models
Moisturizers, α-hydroxy acid-based, 126
Molluscum sebaceum, see Keratoacanthoma
Morphoeic basal cell carcinoma, 77-8
Mottling, 29-30
Mouse model
  hair depigmentation, 49
  solar elastosis, 25-6
Mutations, UV-induced, 62-3

Naevi, see also Basal cell naevus syndrome;
    Melanocytic naevi
Nail plates and aging, 87-8
Nerves, dermal, aging, 90
Neural elements of dermis, aging, 90
Nitric oxide and UV, 100
Nodular melanoma, 41
Nodulocystic basal cell carcinoma, 76-7
Non-Hodgkin's lymphomas and UV, 98
Nuclear retinoid receptors, see Retinoic acid
    receptors; Retinoid X receptors

Occupational outdoor exposure, 3, 7

Oestrogen therapy, menopausal, 139
Oncogenesis, see Carcinogenesis
Onychokygryphosis, 88
Outdoor activities, 7-8
  occupational, 3, 7
Ozone and its destruction, 2, 3-5

Peeling, 126, 132-4
  dyspigmentation, 56-7
  photodysplasia, 79
Phenol peel, 132
Photoaging, see also Solar elastosis
  defined, 11
  intrinsic photoaging compared with, 93-4
  tretinoin use, 121-2
Photoallergy, 104
Photocarcinogenesis, see Carcinogenesis
Photodermatoses, 100-4
Photodysplasia, see Dysplasia
Photographic techniques, 117-18
Photosensitivity, 103-4
Phototoxicity, 103-4
Pigment cells, see Melanocytes
Pigmentary change, 29-60, 112-13
  clinical description, 29-50
    basal cell carcinoma, 35-6, 77
  pathogenesis, 50-1
  treatment, see Treatment
Pigmentation, photodamage related to degree of, 11
Pinch test, 18
Poikiloderma of Civatte, 36-8
Polymorphic light eruption, 101-2
Porokeratosis, disseminated superficial actinic, 71
Premalignant lesions
  for melanoma, 39-41
  for non-melanoma cancer, 37, 64-74
    treatment, 79
Prurigo, actinic, 100
Pseudocolloid millium, 15-16
Pseudoscars, stellate idiopathic, 45-6
Psoralen + UVA, see PUVA
Psoriasiform change
  aging nail plates, 87-8
  Bowen's disease, 71
Purpura, senile, 15, 20
PUVA, as chronic UVR exposure model, 20
PUVA lentigenes, 34

Radiotherapy, lentigo maligna, 40

Raimer's bands, 16
'Red neck', 15
Redness, see Erythema
Rejuvenation surgery, 136
Renal transplantation and skin cancer, 99
Resorcin, 132
Resurfacing
 laser, 134
  dyspigmentation, 56
  photodysplasia, 79
 manual, 134
Reticulated black solar lentigo, 32-3
Retinaldehyde, 125-6
Retinoic acid
 all-*trans*-, see Tretinoin
 13-*cis*-, see Isotretinoin
 pigment cell effects
  cell migration, 53-4
  cell proliferation, 53
  melanogenesis, 52-3
Retinoic acid binding proteins, cellular (CRABP), 54-5
Retinoic acid receptors, 54, 124-5
 retinoid actions, 124-5
Retinoid(s)
 nuclear receptors, see Retinoic acid receptors; Retinoid X receptors
 pigment cell proliferation effects, 53
 topical use, 121-6
  mechanism of action, 124-5
Retinoid X receptors, 54, 124-5
 retinoid actions, 124-5
Retinol binding proteins, cellular (CRBP), 54-5
Rhomboidal furrows, 15
Rhytides, see Wrinkling
Rodent ulcer, see Basal cell carcinoma
Rosacea, 15

'Sailor's skin', 15
'Sallow' skin, 12-13, 112
Scars, stellate, 16
Sebaceous glands
 aging effects, 91
 carcinoma, 78-9
Seborrhoeic keratoses, hyperpigmented, 47-50
Senile comedones, 17-18
Senile keratoses, see Solar keratoses
Senile lentigo, see Actinic lentigo
Senile purpura, 15, 20
SH bonds and solar elastosis, 24

Silicon injection, 127-8
Skin
 cancer, see Cancer
 colour changes, see Colour changes
 peeling, see Peeling
 resurfacing, see Resurfacing
 type, classification, 11, 12
Socioeconomic factors, 7-8
Solar elastosis (solar elastotic degenerative change), 11-25, 114-16
 clinical features, 12-15
 clinical variants, 15-18
 measures, 114-16
  colour changes, 112
 mechanical alterations, 18-21, 116
 models, 25-6
 pathogenesis, 24-5
 pathology, 21-4
 treatment, 26
Solar keratoses (actinic/senile keratoses), 64-70
 clinical features and variants, 66-8
 histopathology, 65-6
 pigmented, 34-5, 68
  spreading, 35
 prevalence/significance, 68-9
Solar lentigo 31-3, 56; Actinic lentigo
Solar purpura, 15, 20
Solar radiation, see Sun
Spreading pigmented actinic keratoses, 35
Squamous cell carcinoma/epithelioma, 74-6
 clinical features, 74-5
 pathology, 75-6
 pigmented, 36
  actinic/solar keratosis and, 35, 69-70
S–S bonds and solar elastosis, 24
Stellate pseudoscars, idiopathic, 45-6
Stellate scars, 16
Stockings, 7
Stratum corneum, age-related change, 86
Suction devices (Cutometer etc.)
 aging skin, 90
 sun-damaged skin, 20, 116
Sulfhydryl bonds and solar elastosis, 24
Summer prurigo, Hutchinson's, 100
Sun (solar stimulus), 1-9
 protection from, 7, 137-8
  from immunosuppressive effects, 104-5
 spectrum/wavelength, 1-3
  photodamage related to, 5-6
Sun worship, 8

Sunscreens (UVA/UVB), 104, 137-8
  in (pre)malignancy prevention, 79
  skin type and, 12
Superficial actinic porokeratosis, disseminated, 71
Superficial basal cell carcinoma, 77
Surgery, 127-30
  aesthetic, 136
  lentigo maligna, 40
  non-melanoma cancer, 79
Sweat glands
  aging effects, 91
  carcinoma, 78-9

T cells (helper T subset) and UV, 99
Telangiectasia in solar elastosis, 13-15, 23
Telomeric shortening, 84
Textiles, 7
TH1/2 cells and UV, 99
Therapy, *see* Treatment
Tocopherol and derivatives, 105, 138
Trabecular carcinoma, 79
Traumatic injury to deeper tissue, aging skin and, 90, 91-2
Treatment, 51-7, 121-42
  chronic actinic dermatitis, 103
  non-melanoma cancer, 79
  photodysplasia, 79
  pigmentary change
    actinic keratosis, 35
    actinic lentigo, *see* Actinic lentigo
    idiopathic guttate hypomelanosis and, 45
    lentigo maligna, 40-1
    measuring effects, 112
    seborrhoeic keratosis, 48
  polymorphic light eruption, 101-2
  skin photoaging/solar elastosis, 26, 121-42
Tretinoin (all-*trans*-retinoic acid), 121-4
  experimental pigment cell studies
    cell migration, 53
    melanogenesis, 53
    retinoic acid receptor studies, 54
  guidelines for use, 123-4
  in hyperpigmentation disorders, 51-2
    depigmenting agents and, 57
    peeling and, 57
  in intrinsic aging, 123
  mechanism of action, 124-5
  in photoaging, 121-2
  in photodysplasia, 9

Triamcinolone, idiopathic guttate hypomelanosis, 45
Trichloracetic acid, 57, 132, 133
Triradiate scars, 16
TRP-1, 49, 53
Tumour suppressing genes, 62, 63
Tyrosinase, retinoic acid effects, 53
Tyrosine-related protein (TRP-1), 49, 53

Ultrasound, solar elastosis, 13, 115-16
Ultraviolet radiation, *see* UV
Urocanic acid, 100
Uronic acid, 89
UV
  as causative factor
    cancer, *see* Carcinogenesis
    idiopathic guttate hypomelanosis, 44-5
    solar elastosis, 11, 24, 25
    solar keratosis, 69
  chronic exposure, model, 20
  as component of solar spectrum, 1-2
  immune response to, 63, 97-107
  melanocyte effects, 50
  protection from, *see* Sun; Sunscreens
UVA
  damaging effect, 5-6
  psoralen +, *see* PUVA
  solar, 1-2
  sunscreens, *see* Sunscreens
  synergism with UVB, 5
UVA lentigenes, 33
UVB
  melanocyte effects, 50
  solar, 2
    diurnal/seasonal variations, 3
    ozone absorbing, 4-5
  sunscreens, *see* Sunscreens
  synergism with UVA, 5
UVC, solar, 2
  ozone absorbing, 2, 3-4

van Gieson's stain, 21, 24, 115
Vasculature, *see* Blood vessels
Verhoeff's stain, 24
Versican, 89
Visual analogue scale, 117
Vitamin C, 105, 138-9
Vitamin E and derivatives (tocopherols), 105, 138

Warty skin tumours, diagnosis, 69

White macules, idiopathic guttate hypomelanosis, 43-4
Whitening of hair, *see* Hair
Wound healing and aging, 91-3
Wrinkling (rhytides), 12
  treatments
    botulinum toxin for glabellar folds, 137
    facelift (rhytidectomy), 136
    laser skin resurfacing, 135-6

Yellow–brown discoloration, 12-13, 112

'Zebra fibres', 24
Zyderm and Zyplast, 128-9